Throughout the ages, God has gone to great lengths to write His story, upon the hearts of all humanity. Ed Williamson's *No Other Name* reveals the heart, mind and soul of one who has discovered God's great story and whose life is shaped by the work of a Holy God. The book is warm and powerful, an inspiring expression of the author's own journey of faith through love, struggle and triumph. It offers a stirring challenge to look for God in every circumstance and He will be found.

Dr. Sandra C. Gray
President, Asbury University
Wilmore, KY

This book is a must-read for anyone facing a physical challenge or who has a loved one dealing with a health issue. I love the balance of the book in terms of faith, medicine, relationships and Scripture. The agony, joy, pain, hopes and expectations are felt as Ed and Loretta deal with her battle with cancer. Most of all, their love for Christ, love for people, and their passion for ministry is felt throughout this insightful book.

Dr. Stan Toler
General Superintent Emeritus
Church of the Nazarene
Oklahoma City, OK

I met Ed and Loretta in a season when Loretta was cancer free following a miraculous healing. Ed was serving as evangelist at Camp Sychar in Mount Vernon, Ohio. The night we met, Ed began the message on marriage and Loretta finished it. Their "tag-team" preaching had a profound effect on my life and my understanding of a biblical theology of marriage. This is a story of Ed and his "Battle Maiden" — a triumph of faith, love, surrender, and family.

Dr. John E. Neihof
President, Wesley Biblical Seminary
Jackson, MS

In this moving book, Ed and Loretta Williamson share their love affair with the Gospel of Jesus Christ and with each other, across decades of ministry and a lengthy battle with cancer that finally ended in Loretta's death. Yet their joy in the Lord, and devotion to each other, never died. I highly recommend this unflinching portrayal of faithfulness amid the ravages of terminal cancer. It is testimony and love story wrapped together. Readers will be blessed by the Williamsons' story, and will gain courage for their own journeys as followers of Christ.

Dr. Dana L. Robert
Director, Global Christianity and Mission
Boston University School of Theology

You will be greatly encouraged and strengthened in your faith as you read *No Other Name*. It is a wonderful tribute to the grace, mercy and help that our Lord can send to others who go through times of trouble and deep waters similar to this couple's. You will rejoice and be delighted by the numerous times of blessing in the midst of their battle with each test that came their way. I strongly urge you to read this compassionate book and share a copy with a friend, for this story is one that will edify both those who know the Lord and those who have not yet become part of His family.

Dr. Walter C. Kaiser, Jr.
President Emeritus, Gordon-Conwell Theological Seminary
Author and premier Bible scholar

In the late sixties, I worked in the ghettos of New York City alongside Loretta, my sister Faith, and others and we enjoyed observing Ed and Loretta's courtship. Even though I knew of Loretta's challenge with cancer in later years, during our infrequent visits she masked the gravity of her battle with her positive, upbeat demeanor.

I was not prepared for the range of emotions I experienced as I read this book. It is a love story, as well as a compelling account of the effects of cancer on one family, and you will see how this most dreaded disease impacted each of them. But overriding it all is the story of their rock-solid faith in Jesus Christ and His supremacy over all of life, even life at its worst. Without being "preachy," these pages will inspire you to make Jesus Christ the ultimate pursuit in your life, for there is "no other name."

Sharon Brown Hervold, Former CURE Corps Member
Language Literacy Specialist (Retired)
Gettysburg, PA

Ed and Loretta Williamson share their deepest feelings in her long battle with cancer. A fascinating and heartwarming story of triumphant faith in the Word of God and a mighty Savior!

Dr. Robert E. Coleman
Former Professor, Gordon-Conwell Theological Seminary
Distinguished Professor of Evangelism
Asbury Theological Seminary

The busiest task of a Children's Pastor is recruiting workers. While serving with us in that position, Loretta had her share of filling positions to make the children's ministry effective. However, she didn't recruit staff in the traditional manner. She thought she could pray them in — and pray she did! Over and over God answered her prayers and brought faithful, qualified workers willing and wanting to work with her. She was a Spirit-led servant, not simply in word but in deed. Having her on our team was a spiritual experience for all of us who worked with her. Heaven is a richer place because Loretta is there. One can sense the presence of the Lord while reading this chronicle of her and her family's life and journey together.

Dr. Charles Lake
Founding Pastor, Community Church of Greenwood
Greenwood, IN

Having known the Williamsons since 1989, I was not suprised to see them being obedient to the Lord as they faced Loretta's cancer and the struggles that came with it. As a physician and Christ lover, I always find it refreshing to see realistic faith and medicine working in concert. Many Christians strive to balance the two. The Williamsons invite us to travel with them through their struggles as they prove that, indeed, faith and medicine can and do work beautifully together. We get a glimpse into Loretta's life, which she lived for the glory of His name and the advancement of His kingdom. Indeed, there is no other name but Jesus. This is a story of life as it happened — well worth the reading and one that I thoroughly enjoyed.

M. Reena Varghese, MD
Internal Medicine
Greensboro, NC

In their vulnerability, the Williamsons have shared an every-man's story. They allow us to walk with them through the valley of the shadow of death as they permit God to conquer their fears by using and trusting in the means of grace. All of us have gone through or will go through a life-tragedy — loss of a loved one, a job, friends, dreams, health — yet when all drops away there truly is no other name that stays. The Williamsons practiced grace as God's Word instructs, not as a magic potion, but as refining truth, and they testify that, indeed, He is sufficient for this life and the next.

> *Dr. Carl B. Fliermans*
> *CEO/President, Ecological Microbes Unlimited*
> *Augusta, GA*

In Loretta's own words, "The secret to endurance is to remember that your pain is temporary, and your reward eternal." That is the deep understanding of a person who embraces the admonitions of the Apostle Paul to set our sights on the realities of heaven and remember that we are citizens of heaven. This book is a tearful and joyful reminder of a woman who lived victoriously in the face of death, loving her Lord, loving her family, and loving those the Lord brought into her path. Her life was a blessing, a powerful affirmation of the joy that is promised in a personal relationship with Jesus, and the message of her life continues from the pages of this book.

> *Dr. David Long*
> *Former President, One Mission Society*
> *Greenwood, IN*

This book is a faith expander with a solid biblical base. The love of Christ pours through the pages and reaches deep into the heart of the reader with hope and healing. Immediately the reader is invited into a powerful journey of the transforming presence of Christ in all circumstances.

> *Jo Anne Lyon, Ambassador*
> *General Superintendent Emerita*
> *The Wesleyan Church*
> *Indianapolis, IN*

I wholeheartedly recommend *No Other Name*! My wife and I were alongside Ed and Loretta Williamson for two decades as the miracles recorded in this book took place. I was serving as General Superintendent of the Evangelical Methodist Church when the Williamsons were led of the Lord to join our denomination. In the years that followed, Leona and I were deeply moved, blessed, and challenged to be at our best for our Lord as, time and time again, we witnessed God's marvelous touch on Loretta. This is a story that needs to be told.

> *Rev. Clyde Zehr*
> *Former General Superintendent*
> *Evangelical Methodist Church*

The story of Ed and Loretta Williamson is truly a journey of faith. It begins with a testament to the providence of God in their individual lives, and continues with God's leading them together and into ministry. The account of their journey with Loretta's cancer brings home the truth that God is always there, in sunshine and in shadows, in joy and in sorrow, in life and in death. Their experience becomes our experience. We rejoice with them, we cry with them. Their faith becomes our faith. We come away with the assurance of the words of Peter in Acts 4:12: "Salvation is found in no one else, for there is no other name under heaven given to mankind by which we must be saved."

> *Dr. J. Duane Beals*
> *Professor of Religion (Retired), Bethel College*
> *South Bend, IN*

NO OTHER NAME

One Couple's Story of Living with Cancer

Ed and Loretta Williamson

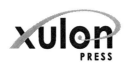

ACKNOWLEDGEMENTS

Special individuals and organizations impacted our story and the writing of the book. The Evangelical Methodist Church family supported us during our journey with cancer, and many individuals encouraged us to continue writing throughout the years.

Our children, Ben, Danielle, and Nathan, gave support and material for the book. Loretta's brother, Armand Dion, and especially her sisters, Bernadette and Denise, assisted in the timeline of events and narrative sections.

The many brothers and sisters in Christ at Asbury University; Asbury Seminary; One Mission Society; Wesley Biblical Seminary; Gordon-Conwell Theological Seminary; and the Global Wesleyan Alliance, who offered to the Lord countless prayers during our journey.

Teen Challenge staff from our CURE Corps days: Shari Hervold, who gave me the incentive to restart working on the book, and Carol Brown Patterson, who made the book a reality.

TABLE OF CONTENTS

FOREWORD

One of the most perplexing issues in the Christian life is what to think about divine healing. Was it just for New Testament times or does it happen today? If so, are today's apparent healings just coincidences? If divine healing does occur today, and it certainly seems to, why doesn't it occur all the time? And why to some people and not others?

This book will not answer all those questions. But it will bring every reader to the realization that our life here on earth is not primarily about maximum physical health, but about a maximally deep relationship with God.

In many ways this book is a love story — the love of Ed and Loretta. But it is even more about the ways in which Loretta's bouts with cancer led both of them to drill down to the depths of their love for God.

Loretta's experiences with cancer ran the gamut: healing by means of medicine; miraculous healing; and, finally, death. In it all were the realities of pain, anger, grief, and uncertainty. Yet, even deeper was the abiding reality of God's love and care, as testified to by His unchanging Word.

As both Loretta and Ed demonstrate, faith is not some magical formula for getting what we want from God. Faith is the unshakeable certainty that God is good, and that if, indeed, His ways are higher than ours, He can be trusted right to the end.

I said at the outset that this book will not answer all our questions about healing. That may be so, but it will answer any question we may have about the power of God to hold His people firm through life's severest storms.

Dr. John N. Oswalt
Visiting Distinguished Professor of Old Testament
Asbury Theological Seminary
Wilmore, KY

DEDICATION

This book is dedicated to our children,
who enriched our lives with their faith and courage.
And to all those families
who are on their own journey with cancer.

Salvation (healing) is found in no one else,
*for there is **no other name** under heaven given to men*
by which we must be saved (Acts 4:12).

PREFACE

"You have cancer."

These words strike fear in the heart and consume enormous amounts of emotional energy, draining the reservoir without providing a replenishing intake. Within a few hours or days of hearing the pronouncement, physical exhaustion emerges with a weariness that has roots deep inside the person. Loretta and I know this to be true, as we have lived it. Death came calling at our door.

This is the story of our personal journey in a battle against a formidable adversary — cancer. We share our personal struggles and reveal emotional upheavals that came as a result of harmful advice given to us by well-intentioned people, as you will see later in the story. Our children share what it was like for them to have their mother's body invaded by cancer and how they dealt with thoughts of her impending death.

We share things that were helpful as well as those that hindered us all during this time in the life of our family. We have tried to be vulnerable and open, yet remain positive and encouraging about the medically verified healing that Loretta experienced after her breast cancer had metastasized to her ribs. A few years later, our world was rocked a second time when a different type of cancer was found in her hip joint. How does this fit into our understanding of God and the Bible?

As pastors, we desire to help people understand that God's presence is with us in sickness and chaos. We also want to demonstrate how one's faith and trust can grow through the intimacy of a personal relationship with Christ, coupled with a saturation of biblical promises. Much that has passed as the Christian ministry of healing is heartless, mindless, and hurtful in its exploitation of people when they are most vulnerable. Healing scriptures are often wrapped in religious jargon rich in emotion but poor in theology. This warps the scriptural intent, offers a false hope to the unsuspecting and vulnerable, and often results in the destruction of lives and the plundering of the spiritual and material well-being of good people.

The opposite of this is a frozen theology of healing that overreacts to the popular excesses, and confines healing only to the days of the twelve apostles. Wrong thinking about healing has become an albatross around the neck of the believer and robs people of experiencing healing through the ministry of the local church. We have experiential, as well as biblical, proof that God heals today, and we attempt to strike a balance between these two extremes. Our goal is to avoid formulas and simply share the practical insights that helped sustain us and move us forward in our faith in God's promises for healing, while heeding medical procedures and advice. Our conviction is that healing is a ministry of the local church.

We begin by sharing about our early days of knowing Christ and how we met on the streets of New York City while working with a ministry to drug addicts called Teen Challenge. We then walk through the story of how this disease, coupled with the traumas of pastoral ministry, almost brought death to Loretta as well as to the ministry. We battled through many emotion-laden memories in writing these pages. Woven throughout are incidents and experiences that illustrate how God worked in our lives.

We share our answers to the barrage of fears and questions we had: "Why, God? Is there sin in our lives? How can God allow sickness and disaster in a world He created and loves? This is not fair!" Our treatment of these topics is not exhaustive, but we present answers that calmed our fears and satisfied our queries. Everything we had ever preached or taught was now being called into play for practical use and living.

The verses and biblical stories that grounded our faith are shared. A recurring theme of the book is that faith is not a frenzied emotion without intellectual moorings to ground it. Faith is relational, not a substance that is injected into the bloodstream or dropped out of heaven through some spiritual IV. Faith and trust find their anchor in the character and integrity of God, nurtured by the conduit of God's Word in the context of an interpersonal relationship with Him.

Jesus is known and believed by many to be a prophet; for instance, He is mentioned 72 times in the Koran. We have found that from the moment of our conception in the womb, God has a specific plan for each one's life — a plan that cannot be fully realized until Jesus transforms us for the journey each has been designed to live.

There is **no other name** but Jesus whereby we are saved and healed (see Acts 4:12). From my vantage point on the platform, I often observed Loretta with her arms lifted in worship and praise to God . . . and in pain. This was especially meaningful when the chorus, *No Other Name*, was being sung. The words to that chorus are reprinted here:

NO OTHER NAME

Words and music by Robert Gay

No other name but the name of Jesus
  No other name but the name of the Lord
No other name but the name of Jesus
  Is worthy of glory, and worthy of honor
And worthy of power and all praise.

CHAPTER 1

LORETTA SPEAKS

Fitchburg, Massachusetts, where I was born, is a paper mill town with a population of approximately 40,000 in the northcentral part of the state. My grandparents settled there, having emigrated from different provinces of Canada, and my parents, Irene and Alphonse Dion, reared us in a strong, French Roman Catholic home.

My two brothers, Armand and George, and two sisters, Bernadette and Denise, and I loved the times when our extended family had big, informal get-togethers. Pépère and Mémère, our French-speaking grandparents, spoke very little English, so we all conversed in French to accommodate them. Occasionally our Mémère Hachey, my mom's mother, told us scary stories about the times Indians attempted to break into their home. She would begin the story in English, get to the tense parts and switch to French, and then conclude in English, unaware of her interchange of the two languages. She was a great storyteller and we kids knew enough French not to miss a beat of the storyline.

My parents were devout and there were several nuns and a priest in our extended family. We children went to parochial school for thirteen years and were well indoctrinated in the tenets of the Catholic Church. We recited the rosary in French while kneeling around the dining room chairs, especially during the Lenten season. We visited shrines to Mary in Canada and said a "Hail Mary" on our knees as we ascended the many steps leading up to the crucifix. By doing this we thought we were earning indulgences for ourselves and any departed loved ones who may still be in purgatory. These exercises were a normal part of my life. We were taught to have respect for God, knowing there were eternal consequences for sins.

In my effort to please God and lead a normal, albeit deeply religious, life, I was cautious, even fearful, and never stepped out of line. In fact, my older sister gave me the title of "Miss Goody Two-Shoes." Sometimes during the summer recess from elementary school, we three older children walked a mile to and from church for early mass. When we arrived home, after a quick breakfast we liked to reenact the mass. My sister played the priest and my brother and I were the "altar boys." We placed oyster crackers in a goblet which we put in the sliding doors of our old player piano. Mass was a very important part of our lives and we recited the entire mass in Latin. When I was in high school, my dad dropped Armand, Bernadette and me off at mass and went on to work; afterward, we walked the mile to school.

My parents made many sacrifices to have all of us in Catholic schools in spite of the financial strain. They felt that God would bless them for putting our education above luxuries.

I was mildly shocked when my sister Bernadette announced that she would be entering the convent as soon as she graduated from high school. She chose a medical missionary order in Pennsylvania, and I knew I wouldn't be able to see her for almost a year. She was a spirited girl, full of life and a little on the wild side, but she desired to be close to God. She thought being a medical missionary would be an adventure and her salvation would be ensured because she was helping people. We had been taught since we were small that total dedication to God meant pursuing a vocation to the priesthood or in a convent.

By temperament I was more suited to the life of a nun than my siblings were. A compliant child, I often ran interference for my sister. When she disappointed our parents, I would tell them that she really didn't mean what she had done. Bernadette went ahead with her plans to enter the convent in September 1963. Our parents always questioned the genuineness of her calling but she seemed determined to demonstrate her sincerity. In fact, when she was home for Easter break, I became concerned for her when I noticed that instead of sleeping on a bed in the room we shared, she was lying on brushes as an act of penance.

And then suddenly in May of 1964 she was sent home, disappointed, humiliated, and thinking that she would probably go to hell. She had believed in a salvation gained by good deeds and building up personal merits to present to God, a "works" gospel, and the convent had been sort of an insurance policy for her — but now that policy was completely torn up. That fall she enrolled in the nursing program at a local state college and I enrolled in the education department, making us freshmen together.

During Bernadette's junior year in college, a young man began to talk to her about Jesus Christ. He also witnessed to several of her friends and they eventually agreed to attend a Bible study, which seemed harmless enough. I had scant knowledge of this at the time, as Bernadette and I were pursuing different degrees and didn't share interests or friends. We caught up with each other only when we were home on holiday.

I was doing student teaching during my senior year when I received a distressing call from my dad about Bernadette. He told me that she desperately needed prayer because she had become involved in some sort of "Jesus Movement" and had gone off the deep end. Returning home at the conclusion of my student teaching, I found my family in the midst of the most trying ordeal in its history.

Bernadette had attended a missions conference sponsored by InterVarsity Christian Fellowship in Urbana, Illinois. John Stott, the guest speaker, presented the gospel out of the book of 2 Timothy and both the speaker and the message had a profound effect on my sister. The truth of the gospel became clear to her and she returned home radically different, excited about what God had done in her life. The conference was not Catholic, which was upsetting in itself, but now she was reading her Bible regularly and quoting it often, much to our parents' dismay. She was spending a lot of time with Denise, our younger sister who was a sophomore at St. Bernard's High School. As a result, Denise was taken by Bern's zeal and began to read the Bible; her life started changing, as well. George, the baby of the family, was a seventh grader and seemed unaffected by it all, and Armand, now in the Air Force in Florida, was also unaffected.

At her Catholic high school, Denise began to tell others about her spiritual awakening, encouraging them to read their Bibles. She was a cheerleader and before long some of the students started yelling, "Repent!" at her during basketball games. Similar comments were made in the halls, and within a few months Denise's best friend

4

confided that her parents would not allow her to be friends with her any longer. The nuns then decided that she could not be in class with the other students and she spent her days in the library in independent study.

During this time, the high school headmaster called our parents in for a conference. After talking with Denise, he had come to the conclusion that she was excessively interested in God for a girl her age. He felt that Dad should explore possibilities of what may have caused such a change in her behavior. You see, it was just fine for us to go to mass every day and say the rosary, but reading the Bible or developing a personal relationship with God sent red flags flying!

Dad asked the parish priest to meet with Denise and "talk some sense into her." When Denise arrived for the appointment, the young assistant priest met with her for several hours. He did most of the talking and at one point he shared that he did not believe that hell existed. She had brought with her a well-worn copy of GOOD NEWS FOR MODERN MAN, a modern translation of the New Testament, and before she left, the priest took it from her. He replaced her Bible with a book about the historical Jesus. This was the late 1960's when Catholics weren't encouraged to read their Bibles except in the presence of a priest, who could interpret it for them. It was also a time of extreme turmoil because of Vatican II, which may have accounted for the priest's strange and radical ideas.

The priest was convinced that Denise had converted to a form of heresy at the behest of Bernadette and he felt that Bernadette should be asked to leave home so that her influence would be removed from the house. He hoped that this course of action would also cause Denise to come to her senses and return to the faith. So my parents asked Bernadette to move out. She was not involved with any particular denomination but had attended a strong Baptist church since accepting Christ and this pastor and his family took her into their home while she looked for an apartment close to the college.

As I had in the past, I became the mediator between Bernadette and my parents, in hopes of reconciliation. My first visit to Bern's apartment wasn't at all what I had anticipated. I had thought maybe she was in a cult and needed to be deprogrammed. She was sweet, soft-spoken, and loving toward me. In other words, she was different; a real change had come over her. It wasn't just that she was nicer than usual, but she was patient and seemed sure of what she was doing and where she was going. I realized that she held no bitterness toward my parents or the priest. Truly, my sister had come to know Jesus in a very personal, powerful way.

As we shared about various things, Bern began to tell me that she had traded religion for a relationship with God. She explained that she had spent her whole life trying to please God, when, in fact, there was nothing she could do to earn His love. As she shared with me about God's love demonstrated by Christ's sacrificial death on the cross, I sensed that these were new revelations to her. A change had come over her after she attended the InterVarsity Christian Fellowship conference. She made it clear to me that the gospel was not realized by being baptized into the Church but by faith alone in Christ's work on the cross. This was all new to me. She quoted Bible verses and gave me a paperback copy of the New Testament, encouraging me to read it. I informed her that our parents weren't sleeping at night because of her and chided her for her radical beliefs. Yet, when I left her I told her that I would be back.

At home I was able to observe my younger sister, Denise, and the subtle changes in her life. She had been a typical teenager: a smart, popular cheerleader and a science scholar. In fact, I think that she and George were the most intellectual of the five of us, always excelling in their schoolwork. When I asked Denise if I could borrow a sweater from her, she graciously responded that I could borrow any of her clothes I wanted. This would never have been her response in the past. Her countenance was similar to Bern's and I was beginning to think that there might be something to this Jesus "cult" that was influencing them. I understood why my parents had asked Bern to leave, as she had definitely strongly influenced Denise. I certainly didn't find fault with Denise's behavior, but I just felt it wasn't normal for a fifteen-year-old.

I continued to visit Bern but decided that the best way to deal with her was to meet her on her "territory." I would read the Bible and try to prove to her that she was misinterpreting it. I was determined to fight fire with fire! So my visits to Bern's apartment continued mainly so I could argue with her and win her back to normalcy. Sometimes I felt as though I was making real progress, but other times I would leave completely frustrated. I was concerned, as she and I were in our last semester of college. I was working twenty hours each week for the chairperson of the Special Education Department, while Bern was working many more hours at a local nursing home just to make ends meet. There wasn't much time to "win her back" and I wasn't making much progress. When I thought I had a good argument, she would show me what the Word said. After three months of this, I realized that Bern wasn't attempting to convert me to a particular movement or denomination, but just to the Word of God, the Bible.

On March 13, 1968, as I peppered her with questions, Bern took me through a little booklet entitled, *The Four Spiritual Laws*. It provided a simple explanation of why Christ had to die and how we could know Him personally. It ended with the question, "Is there any reason why you can't trust in Him today for your salvation?" My response was a simple, "No."

I realized that after all my arguments, my problem was not with Bernadette, but rather with the Word of God. I hadn't been sure that I could trust the Bible if it contradicted some of my beliefs but the Holy Spirit opened my eyes. Now, that had changed and I told her that I was ready to repent of my rebellion to God's Word and put my faith and trust in Him. I prayed a simple prayer with my sister and then returned home.

It was not until the next day that I realized the change in my life. There were early signs of spring all around and as I observed the budding crocuses, I began to recognize the signs of my new life with Christ: a sense of His presence and a peace I had never realized. I had known Him in a reverent, worshipful way before, but now I knew that He loved me and died on the cross just for me. The next Sunday I attended mass with the family and the Scriptures took on a life with true meaning for the first time. When I read the Bible, it was as though the letters were written personally to me; the words of Jesus seemed directed just to me. I developed a strong desire to read the Bible for the first time, finding it relevant to my life.

I was teaching catechism on Wednesday nights to high school students and I recall telling them about my conversion experience. I wanted to let these kids know how relevant the Word was for their needs. It had not yet occurred to me that I wouldn't remain a Catholic. I assumed that I would just be a better one and would help others of that faith discover how the Bible could help them come to know Jesus better.

Denise soon saw the change in my life and our relationship became closer and richer. She told me she had won school friends to the

Lord and given Bibles to them. Bernadette and her friends were happy to supply the Bibles. We began to pray for our parents and asked the Lord for opportunities to talk to them calmly about what God had done in our lives. We were able to have some good one-on-one conversations with them, which were then often followed by times of anger and hostility. I decided to keep a low profile to avoid suffering the same fate as Bernadette. Denise, on the other hand, became much bolder in sharing her new faith with Mom and Dad.

My dad, only about forty-two years old at the time, experienced a bout of thrombophlebitis (a blood clot in the leg). He was taking a blood thinner for this, as well as using a heating pad to dissolve the clot. One evening Denise asked Dad if he would believe what the Bible said if he observed a healing.

"What do you mean?" Dad replied.

"Well, I've been telling you about God's power to save and to heal. If God healed your leg, would that verify the truth of the Bible for you?"

When Dad replied that it might, Denise gave him instructions and made a bold claim. "Stop taking your medication and don't use the heating pad. God is going to completely heal your leg during the night. I can assure you of this because the Word of God is true."

Dad reluctantly agreed to do as she asked, thinking it would cause her to come to her senses when she saw that God doesn't do that anymore, except in rare instances.

The next morning Denise greeted him with, "It's gone, isn't it, Dad? Your leg is healed, isn't it?" The blood clot, in fact, was gone and the doctor verified it at Dad's next appointment. I was in awe of Denise's faith. Still, Mom and Dad continued to resist.

A few weeks after my conversion, Denise and I were watching a Billy Graham Crusade on television while our parents were out for the evening. At some point during his signature altar call, we realized that George had watched the entire program. He was only twelve years old at the time and had been quietly affected by what had been going on around him. He cried as he told us that what the preacher said made sense to him and he wanted to ask Christ into his life. Denise and I led him in a prayer. We all cried together, as this made three committed Christians in the home.

I gave George my Bible since Bern had given me a nice new one. His was much like the one he had seen Billy Graham hold up while he was preaching. We were able to watch the televised crusade that entire week, as our parents were away each evening. At the end of the week I caught George standing in front of a mirror with a Bible in one hand, pretending to preach. I laughed and asked him why he was preaching. He replied that he thought that someday God would use him to bring life back to a cold church by preaching the truth of His Word.

Our parents continued to disapprove and the final straw came when Denise and George devised a Bible verse "treasure hunt" one morning while Mom and Dad were attending early mass. The plan was that when they returned home, they would see a verse on the front door (a "clue") telling them where the next verse was located. We hoped they would follow these Bible verses until they reached the last clue, where they would find Denise and George praying for their salvation. This is not the way it played out, however. Mom and Dad became angry, blamed the scheme on me, and offered me the same ultimatum they had given to Bern four months earlier.

After their outburst of anger, I went upstairs to pray and ask God what I should do. I randomly opened my Bible and this is the verse that came up:

> *"If any man comes to me, and hate not his father, and mother, and wife, and children, and brethren, and sisters, yea, and his own life also, he cannot be my disciple"* (Luke 14:26, KJV).

I knew what the Lord was asking of me. I must be willing to stand for Him even if it meant losing my family.

The harder part was yet to come. I had to stand before my dad and tell him what he did not want to hear. He interpreted my choice as choosing Bernadette and Paul (the young man who had led Bern to the Lord) over him. He could not see that I was following God's Word and was not a part of a deceptive cult. He cried and stated that he would rather be told that I had cancer than to be told that I had left the faith I was reared in. He was still crying when Bern and Paul arrived to pick me up, holding the one suitcase that I had quickly packed. I will never forget the pain in my dad's eyes as I left. I was the one child who never disappointed him or gave him trouble, and I was inflicting a wound that seemed mortal.

When I got to the apartment, Bern offered me some freshly baked brownies, a little hard from overbaking but a gracious gesture on her part. We quickly adapted to our meager lifestyle and were determined to share our faith with our friends. It had been a well-kept secret for too long.

We were just about eight weeks from graduation when I had a short visit with my mom on a trip home to collect the last of my belongings. She remonstrated that this new faith might be fine for me now, but if a serious problem were to arise, it would not be strong enough to sustain me. I reflected on this, and then prayed to God to demonstrate for Mom that this was simply not the case. Three days later I was called into the school office and informed that I was lacking three credits to graduate. I had dropped a subject my freshman year which I had neglected to make up, and the deficit was just now showing up on my records. I realized that God was giving me something to trust Him with. Half the semester was over and my parents thought I might flunk out, as they had been told that I was spending all my time in Bible studies. If I could find a way to make up these credits, I felt that would confirm to them that I was not following a pied piper and had not been trapped and misled.

I prayed and asked the Lord to rescue me and then I went to work. I typed a proposal for the head of my department telling him about my plight with the missing class. He stated that since I was a student in good standing, he would ask the professor to allow me admission to the class at that late date. There would be make-up work to complete, with lots of reading, but he thought it was doable. This meant that I would be carrying twenty hours of course work. In addition, I had been awarded a grant to do research in special education and was in the middle of doing a major paper for that. However, God did, indeed, rescue me and I received a 4.0 grade average that semester. I was still able to share Christ and have Bible studies in our apartment, all the while keeping up my studies.

The Bible studies in our apartment were held on Friday nights and Bern and I invited friends with whom we had been sharing Christ. Afterwards we always offered some refreshments. We had one white enamel pan, the perfect size for a single-layer Jiffy cake, which we would bake and ice to serve.

"Let's pray that today will be someone's spiritual birthday and this will be their birthday cake," Bern suggested one evening. And every time we did this someone accepted Christ.

One day it dawned on us that we were limiting God, so we bought another pan and prepared two cakes, believing for two first-time believers. It happened that night that two of our friends came to trust Christ as their savior! Never had religion brought us this much joy. Oh, there were challenges and difficulties, but the peace of knowing that we were in the center of God's will was overwhelming.

One of our greatest concerns continued to be our parents, including their restrictions on visits from George and Denise. Their Bibles were taken from them and they were never left in the house alone for fear that they might talk and encourage one another in their "deception." We had to place them in God's hands.

Bern and I both graduated from college with honors and I secured a teaching position in a community near Cape Cod. I rented a small beach cottage, which the owners rented to teachers in the fall after they had used it during the summer for their family fun. I taught there only one school term but I realized that as much as I loved teaching, I wanted to offer the students more than just math, reading and the usual curricula. I wanted to offer them Christ. I began to visit various missions conferences and crusades, wondering all the while how Protestant women received a call from God. Was there a Protestant convent or was missions my only option?

In the meantime, Bern married Paul in a bittersweet ceremony. Although my parents attended the wedding, Dad would not give Bern away to Paul, the man responsible for "stealing" his whole family from him. This didn't bode well for me, as I was just about to tell them that I was leaving my wonderful, secure teaching position to go into a form of full-time Christian ministry (something they had prayed for). However, it would not take me into a convent, as they had hoped, but rather to a Christian drug rehabilitation program called Teen Challenge in New York City.

I first heard of Teen Challenge when Bern and I attended a service at a Baptist church in our hometown. David Wilkerson, the speaker, gave a forceful presentation and my sister and I felt compelled to respond to the altar call. We were privileged to speak to him personally and share some of our story. He prayed over us and then quoted the verse from Acts 16:31: "Believe on the Lord Jesus Christ, and thou shalt be saved, and thy house."

I could not have imagined that later I would be an extra in a movie of Mr. Wilkerson's ministry to gang members in New York City. *The Cross and the Switchblade* film included a climactic scene depicting the dramatic conversion of Nicky Cruz (Erik Estrada) at the end of a sermon by David Wilkerson (Pat Boone) and I was one of the extras sitting in the pews.

In my first year of teaching on Cape Cod, someone gave me a copy of the news magazine published by Teen Challenge, and I learned that they were forming a new urban ministry called CURE Corps (Collegiate Urban Renewal Effort). This was David Wilkerson's Christian version of the Peace Corps, which was launched during President John F. Kennedy's administration. The goal was to penetrate an urban area with helping hands, accompanied by the offer of hope through Christ to families who had been devastated by drugs and crime.

I immediately applied to join the original staff, even though it meant giving up my teaching job, and was accepted. God has such a sense of humor. I was the child who was not on the wild side, the cautious one, the one riddled with fears of going on my own to the big city. And now, fearful, cautious "Miss Goody Two-Shoes" was going to be working with drug addicts.

Just as I was getting ready to purchase a bus ticket to the city, Dad offered to drive me there, knowing my determination to go. It seemed foolish to him that I had just sold my new green Volkswagen Bug, and he wouldn't rest until he saw where this reckless daughter was going in her attempt to follow God. It was arranged that my parents, along with George and Denise, would take me and then do some vacationing before returning home.

We arrived at the neighborhood in Brooklyn where the female workers were housed and it seemed safe enough. Shari Brown, a staff worker, met us and assisted me in getting settled. After my parents left, Shari and I drove up to the Bronx, which would be my mission field for the next two years. I recall that hot, muggy August evening as we rode though Brooklyn, over the Brooklyn Bridge into Manhattan, and up FDR Drive to the Willis Avenue Bridge. Crossing over this bridge brought us into the South Bronx …and onto Fox Street.

We were greeted by the distinctive Latin beat of Puerto Rican music and the unmistakable aroma of their cuisine: peppers and onions, exotic spices, and beer. I later learned that this street housed mostly Puerto Ricans and Blacks.

It was difficult for Shari to navigate up the block, as the streets were lined with double- and triple-parked cars. Overflowing trash cans spilled out into the streets, mixing their fetid odor with the more pleasant aromas of ethnic cooking. This street alone was home to roughly 4,000 people and God had led our director,

David Wilkerson, to open a storefront as a ministry center to the neighborhood.

That evening the street meeting consisted of our showing a film about Teen Challenge. The staff set up a projector and screen on the sidewalk and people crowded into the street to catch a glimpse of the film. We had to closely guard our equipment in case a drug addict decided to steal it to finance his next fix. That evening I experienced the wonderfully exhilarating sensation of being "home." I was discovering that, for the child of God, home is being in the center of His will, wherever that might be.

I grew to love my co-workers, who came from many different areas of the country and from a variety of church backgrounds, each answering the call of God on his/her life. Most of us were recent college graduates who had heard about David Wilkerson's ministry among gangs and drug addicts, as well as his highly publicized and well-attended youth crusades of the sixties.

We initially rented one storefront, then two, and finally three on Fox Street in the South Bronx. We started a preschool and offered it to the families at minimal charge. Because we loved their children, they gradually began to trust us, and we were allowed to come into their homes and have Bible studies.

In the late afternoons the preschool was converted into a clubhouse for school-age children. We wanted them to experience the love of God in their early youth because we knew that as they learned to trust Christ to fill the void in their hearts, they would be equipped to circumvent the destruction of drug addiction. Over time, trust in us extended to the addicts on the block. It was beautiful to see how they looked out for our safety, recognizing that God had sent us. They never would have physically harmed us or allowed anyone else to, but they would rob us at the drop of a hat, so addictive were their drug habits.

Shortly after I settled into life with CURE Corps, I received a letter from my mom telling me that my dad had suffered a heart attack and was in the Intensive Care Unit at one of our hometown hospitals. She implied that his worry over me had caused him immense stress and had contributed to his attack. I was deeply concerned, of course, and prayed even harder for him. A few days later I received a letter from Dad stating that while he was recovering, he had read *The Cross and the Switchblade*, written by David Wilkerson. He said it had really touched his heart, and he believed that God was leading me.

What a difference a few days made! I had been held responsible for my dad's heart attack, and now God was using his crisis to get his attention through reading about the ministry I was involved with. I was beginning to learn that God uses everything, even crises, if we're willing to trust Him and rely upon Him. That was the start of the healing in my parents' hearts. They invited me home that Christmas, even offering to pay my bus fare. After all, my salary was only a meager $35 a week, plus room and board.

During my two years with CURE Corps, God taught me many lessons, not the least of which is that programs, or even a sincere heart, cannot transform a drug addict. The thing that transforms an addict is the power of the gospel of Jesus Christ.

> *"I am not ashamed of the gospel, because it is the **power** of God that brings salvation to everyone who believes"* (Romans 1:16).

Our government had invested a large amount of money in methadone, a substitute drug created to help addicts kick their habits. Methadone had a proven cure rate of only 6 percent. Then the government did a comprehensive study of "addicts" from Teen Challenge. They followed them for up to twelve years after their graduation from the program, and were astounded to find that Teen Challenge's cure rate was 86 percent. They labeled the reason for this astounding cure rate THE JESUS FACTOR.

After I returned from a vacation with my family, my ministry partner, Faith Brown, asked me to join her on a short jaunt to Long Island to visit her sister, Carol Patterson, and her family. When we arrived back at the Brooklyn Teen Challenge Center, Faith and I encountered a young man, Ed Williamson, who had just driven into town. He was able to arrange an impromptu interview with Don Wilkerson, Director of the Center, and relate to him how God had moved in a supernatural way on his campus, Asbury College in Wilmore, Kentucky. (Asbury College became Asbury University on March 5, 2010.) He followed up by telling Pastor Don that he knew he had been called to New York City.

Since Pastor Don had heard of the awakening on the Asbury campus, he invited Ed to join the team of CURE Corps workers . . . that very day. I was skeptical, afraid that he would be an idealistic, "here today, gone tomorrow" type of individual and not benefit our cause much. We had had a few of these. But the next day he showed up on the block where we were working and began ministering to the youngsters alongside us.

We were all grateful to have another male on the team. Several young men had come for the initial year of the ministry and had served faithfully, but most had left to return to other commitments once their year was complete. We needed strong role models for the young boys on the block whose older brothers were into the drug scene.

Ed jumped right in, doing anything his skills were called for: changing and/or rotating tires; keeping the oil changed in the vehicles; taking the van into the shop when needed. He was a real team player, willing and cheerful. The thing that impressed me most about him was his belief that nothing was impossible for God, which was vital in a work often characterized by hopelessness. He brought a fresh sense of excitement to what we were doing. I recall that he encouraged us to fast as a team on our days off so that we might see some real "breakthrough" in the lives of those we were working with.

There had been no dating among the members of CURE Corps, not because of any rules but because it just hadn't happened. Some of the workers were in relationships outside of our tight-knit group, but I was not in a relationship at the time; actually, I sometimes wondered if I would ever marry. I was very careful not to let my emotions get away from me with this nice-looking and helpful new recruit.

Slowly I found myself really liking this guy's heart for the Lord in spite of my resolve not to get emotionally involved. Mary, one of our teammates, said that she thought Ed "liked" me. To this I replied, "No way!" He was cordial and gracious to everyone and he was four years younger than I (he had just turned twenty and I was a mature twenty-four-year-old). I had always dated older fellows and planned to follow that precedent. As we all worked together as a team, I enjoyed watching him interact with the youngsters. When he offered hope in Christ to a drug addict, he did so with such love and commitment to the individual. I really did love Ed as a brother in Christ.

One weekend, Ed suggested that the team go to a stock car race out on Long Island. We were supposed to gather in front of the Teen

Challenge Center but only Ed and I showed up. I suddenly faced a personal dilemma. I wasn't sure I should go, as I didn't want it to look like a date, but then I recalled what Mary had told me and I certainly didn't want to disappoint Ed.

Ed and I decided to go ahead and drive on out to the track. We got lost along the way and after we finally arrived we found out that the last race of the season had occurred the previous weekend. We took advantage of our time alone as we drove back to Brooklyn and just talked and talked and talked, sharing and learning about each other. We drove around for several hours and then stopped in a parking area under the Verrazano-Narrows Bridge. Ed told me that this was the exact spot he had come to when he entered the city and asked God for direction. And then he leaned over and kissed me. Fireworks exploded! My time of denial was over — I was in love with this guy and he with me. He later told me that he believed from the moment he met me that we would be in ministry together as life partners, but he had never shared that with anyone or tried to "win" me.

We met in August 1970 and were married in May 1971. My mother claims that he was an answer to her prayers, but in her prayers she forgot to ask for a "good Catholic boy." Nonetheless, my family also fell in love with Ed.

CHAPTER 2

ED'S CALL

~•~

West Virginia is home to me. My father's father, Moses Williamson, emigrated from Ireland through New Jersey to Virginia (now West Virginia) and my mother was from Scots-Irish and Welsh (English) ancestry. Both my parents grew up on farms, although my paternal grandfather was also involved in gas and oil wells in Texas and West Virginia.

My grandfathers and several uncles, as well as Dad, served in World War I and World War II, creating a patriotic extended family. My father loved post-World War II millwright work but working at it meant that we moved frequently. In fact, we moved several times when I was in the first grade, from Baltimore, MD, to Cincinnati, OH, to Parkersburg, WV. We lived in trailer parks and every move meant encountering a new "pecking order" among the boys in the park. This always involved some sort of "fight" and as the oldest of three children, I often found myself protecting my sister.

After years of moving, when I was in the seventh grade my mother told my dad that moving the family from job to job must stop. So we returned to Parkersburg and in the following years we engaged in what could be referred to as "barn raising" — erecting homes and buildings for uncles and aunts. During this time I developed carpentry skills that I was able to use to support my family and work my way through seminary.

My daily routine in childhood included a half-mile walk down a dusty, gravel road to the bus stop. My parents were committed to the Christian faith and instilled biblical values in my brother, sister and me. The grace of God drew me to salvation when I was twelve years old, and at age fourteen I received a clear call from God to His service. However, I ran from entering the ministry and a year following my high school graduation, I made up my mind to enlist in military service and serve in Vietnam. I went to the recruiting office on a Friday afternoon only to learn that the recruiter was on a lunch break, so I returned home planning to go down again on Monday. But that Sunday God renewed His call on my life. He cleansed my heart of all resistance to His calling and replaced it with a passion for His will for my life.

I was accepted into Asbury College in August 1969 just before the opening academic quarter. The dean accepted me on "academic probation" based on my high school records. God has a sense of humor because twenty-five years later I served on the Board of Trustees of this wonderful Christian liberal arts university that helped shape my life and worldview.

During my first academic quarter at Asbury, I read several Christian biographies in addition to my assigned class reading.

Fellow students began discussing a book entitled *The Cross and the Switchblade* that was making the rounds on campus and were excited that the author, David Wilkerson, was going to be speaking in Lexington soon. I read the book and joined a group to hear Reverend Wilkerson preach and share about God's work through the expanding ministry of Teen Challenge.

During a regular chapel service conducted in Hughes Auditorium in February 1970, God flooded our campus with His presence. A student went to the front and told the student body that he felt a need to confess sin, and soon other students followed. Students were joined by professors, all confessing sins and being reconciled to one another. Thus began a miraculous move of God on our campus. Classes were cancelled as students and professors sought God for seven days and nights. By the weekend only a few of the one thousand students were left on campus, as most had returned to their home churches to share their experiences. Everywhere testimonies were given, a similar visitation of God occurred in the congregation.

Throughout that week I felt the Holy Spirit impress on my heart that I was to go to New York City for ministry. Many thought that my emotions had gotten the best of me and my leading might be more of a pipe dream than a call from God. Yet, I recognized God's voice as clearly as when I had experienced my initial call to ministry and I continued to seek the Lord the remainder of that quarter. I spent much of the summer traveling around the country with a singing group, sharing what God had done during that special week of what has become known as the "1970 Revival." (Read *One Divine Moment* by Robert E. Coleman.)

Instead of returning to school the following fall, I packed my bags and said good-bye to my family to follow what had become a real passion in my soul. My parents were somewhat reluctant to allow me to go to the big city with no housing or tangible means of support. Yet, they recognized that this was God's leading, so they prayed with me and sent me on with their blessing.

I had no contacts in New York City whatsoever, but I strongly believed that God would make my path clear. Here I was, a nineteen-year-old boy from West Virginia, facing life in a major metropolis for the first time. After I entered the city, I came to the Verrazano-Narrows Bridge that connects the boroughs of Staten Island and Brooklyn. I pulled over under the bridge to seek God and once again I asked Him to guide me. As I prayed over the city with a heavy burden for the people living there, God's peace enveloped me.

I drove on into Brooklyn and encountered many turns and intersections, not totally sure of where I was going, yet confident that God was guiding me. Before long I looked up and saw a street sign that read "Clinton Avenue," which I recognized as the street that Teen Challenge was on. I turned onto the street and soon found 444 Clinton Avenue, the address of the Brooklyn Teen Challenge Center. After parking my car on the street, I entered the building and encountered a pretty young woman with long, dark hair, wearing knee-high boots and a green dress, walking across the lobby. I later learned that she was Loretta Dion, one of their valued workers.

The receptionist welcomed me and then engaged me in conversation after I asked if I could speak with either David or Don Wilkerson. I related much of the Asbury College story to her, wanting to validate my interest in Teen Challenge. Reverend Don Wilkerson agreed to talk to me and in his office I shared with him about the revival on the Asbury campus and my call to ministry in the city. He had read about the revival and welcomed my first-hand testimony. He then offered me a temporary assignment to work with CURE Corps, a new ministry begun the previous year by his brother, David, to reach the youth of the ghettos before their lives became ravished by sin. CURE Corps had just completed its first year and several of its volunteers had returned home, having fulfilled their year's commitment. New recruits were needed and I was eager to begin.

I became the third male on a team of seven young people who traveled from Brooklyn to Fox Street in the Bronx where the ministry office and preschool were located. Two team members, in particular, figured in my life: Faith Brown and Loretta Dion. Faith had been a charter member, one of the first recruits the previous year, and now had a leadership role in the ministry. She and Loretta worked as a team and I followed their lead because they knew the people, the community, and the heart of the ministry.

It was a real "ride" having Faith drive the van across Brooklyn up to the Bronx, with Loretta leaning out the passenger side window, smiling and flashing those big brown eyes at the drivers to persuade them to allow us to "cut" in front of them. But it worked every time!

On my first visit to Fox Street in the Bronx, I was brought to tears as I saw the youth and children running up and down the street alongside as many as two hundred drug addicts. I had heard about such things but seeing it firsthand always brought a lump to my throat.

The CURE Corps staff had told me about the shooting galleries, places where addicts injected heroin into their veins. We regularly visited Fox Street and the residents became accustomed to our presence. One day we noticed the addicts scattering as we drove onto the block, which was highly unusual, as they usually greeted us. Anyway, this particular day we didn't seem welcome so we inquired about it. We were reminded that the day before as we had walked up and down the sidewalk, we had touched and prayed for the addicts who were so high that the cigarettes they were holding were burning the flesh on their fingers. So what had happened? Well, the users had instantly lost their "high" and they told the other addicts not to let us pray over them or they would waste their high. No wonder they weren't glad to see us coming.

During this time an NYPD officer from Brooklyn contacted Loretta and Faith and asked them to meet him at a local diner. He had heard of the success of Teen Challenge in working with drug addicts and there was someone he wanted them to meet. On a cold, wintry evening the three of them met and sat at a window table. The officer pointed to Maria, who was just across the street getting ready for a night of engaging in prostitution.

He wondered if Loretta and Faith would be willing to offer her some help and, of course, they were eager to get involved. They went directly across the street and talked to Maria, who was addicted to heroin. She was hesitant to talk with them because they were interfering with her "business" but they were able to get some of her story and also share the love of Christ with her. Her boyfriend was in jail and she was working the streets in order to get money for her addiction. Soon, Faith had to leave for an appointment and Loretta continued talking with Maria. In fact, Maria's pimp got angry at Loretta because Maria expressed such interest in the gospel. In time, Loretta was able to give Maria a Bible and set up a time for her to meet for a Bible study.

Following four weeks of Bible study with Loretta and Faith, Maria believed in Christ for the forgiveness of her sins and was radically transformed. She entered the Teen Challenge program for women and was doing exceptionally well. However, just two months before Loretta and I were married, Maria was drawn away from the program by her boyfriend, who had been released from jail. She tried to witness to him about Christ, but as so often happens to young Christian girls, her unsaved boyfriend lured her back to a drug-filled lifestyle. When we left New York City, Maria was back on the streets, more enslaved than ever.

Incidentally, ten years later Loretta and I accompanied a youth group to visit Teen Challenge in New York. Just as we exited our car in Lower Manhattan for a worship service, we heard a loud, shrill cry, "Loretta! Loretta!" Turning, we saw Maria running toward us. She shared how God had lovingly drawn her back to Him and cleansed her from drugs . . . and all her sinning. She had come for the service and as the congregation sang out the chorus, *Our God Reigns,* we were able to watch Maria. Dressed in a beautiful white dress, and with tears streaming down her cheeks, she raised her hands in worship to her Savior. It was a glorious sight! Surely, God does reign and He answers prayer. Maria had been on our prayer list during those many years and we had wondered if we would ever see her again.

I must have passed muster with the others on the CURE Corps ministry team, because within a few weeks they informed Reverend Wilkerson that they would welcome me into their ranks. Later in life, Loretta pointed back to my being accepted and brought on board so quickly. She recalled that she had had to fill out a detailed application, go through an interview, then wait for a call of acceptance while I waltzed in sans all that and went right to work. In fact, it was weeks before she had received an acceptance call . . . and instead of calling her apartment, they had called her parents' house. So they had to relay to her the information that she had been accepted into the Teen Challenge ministry.

As Loretta and I worked together on the streets, we grew to love each other. I remember having some guilt over my growing feelings and I walked around Brooklyn late at night telling God that I didn't come to New York to acquire a girlfriend or a wife. Loretta began to develop romantic feelings for me, as well, but carefully kept them hidden. As I reflect on that beginning phase of our relationship, I see that what drew us to one another was the single-minded passion for serving the Lord and following His will, regardless of the cost.

Although Loretta and I worked diligently at being discreet about our feelings for each other, it wasn't lost on one of the precocious preschool children. This little girl called Loretta by a pet name, Soloretta, and one day she told her mom with a delighted giggle, "Mommy, I heard Pastor Ed call Teacher Soloretta honey!" From then on the word was out all over Fox Street.

Loretta and I marveled at how God had sovereignly brought us together. She had graduated from Fitchburg State University and was teaching on Cape Cod when God called her to work in New York City. God led me from West Virginia to Asbury College in Kentucky where He poured out His Spirit in a great revival and called me to New York City. What might have appeared as small, insignificant decisions at the moment turned out to be acts of obedience that brought two of His children together for forty-two years (we were married on May 8, 1971, in Brooklyn, New York).

—

CHAPTER 3

OUR EARLY YEARS

After our marriage, Loretta and I returned to Asbury College and she stayed busy with her teaching career in special education while I pursued my undergraduate degree. We had hoped to begin our family during this time but there were difficulties that required the intervention of medical specialists. Toward the end of those three years, Loretta did become pregnant and when we received the positive pregnancy report, we were so overcome with joy that we knelt by the couch in our apartment and offered prayers of gratitude. Right then we committed our firstborn child to the Lord.

We left for Gordon-Conwell Theological Seminary in Massachusetts after my graduation from Asbury College in 1974 and Benjamin was born in Beverly (just north of Boston) as I entered seminary.

After completing work on my master's degree at GCTS in 1976, I wanted to complete a second master's at Asbury Theological Seminary in order to study under specific professors whom I believed could help shape me and my ministry. During this time of study, our only daughter, Danielle, was born in Lexington, Kentucky.

After graduating from Asbury Seminary in 1978, I received a pastoral appointment with the United Methodist Church in North Central West Virginia between Fairmont and Morgantown. We entered our first pastorate with Danielle in a body cast to correct a congenital hip joint dislocation. There were frequent trips to Shriners Hospital in Lexington, Kentucky, to replace the cast and check her progress. We enjoyed six years of fruitful ministry here before God led us to go in a new direction.

In 1984 we moved to Morgantown and planted Covenant Evangelical Methodist Church, meeting in the local Ramada Inn. We poured our hearts and lives into this, our first full pastorate, and over the next fourteen years we established a church that launched five daughter churches. Our third baby, Nathan, was born not long after our move to Morgantown.

One day while driving home after a day of ministry, I suddenly sensed God speaking to my heart. He showed me that even though I was faithfully serving Him in this small church, in my heart I was planning to move on to something bigger within a few years. After all, I had two master's degrees and felt that I could do better.

God went right to work on me and began to cleanse the pride and arrogance from my heart. And immediately I knew I was to serve this people as if they were the only congregation I would ever serve. Entering the parsonage, I saw Loretta standing at the kitchen sink. When she heard me, she turned and I saw that she was crying.

"Ed," she said, "God just touched my heart and said that we are to serve Him here as if we will be here for our entire ministry." What a confirmation from the Lord. What a wife and teammate!

When our children were still quite small, Loretta had a dream about the persecution of Christians. She saw a vivid picture of our children and realized later that the Lord was speaking to her heart about preparing them for their walk with Him. She determined to provide them with a strong foundation in the Word of God and impart knowledge about the spiritual battles that face Christians. Her study on spiritual warfare included having Nathan draw pictures of what the lesson said since he could not yet read. In an unexpected blessing, this might have been preparation for her future battle with cancer.

Loretta's vision for our children and others, as well as her education, propelled her into establishing a fine Christian school, Covenant Christian School, in 1990.

Even as we worked tirelessly at serving, training and loving our congregation, we were intent on bringing up our children in the knowledge of Christ. We grappled with the challenges common to all parents and sought the wisdom of God. Every summer we had a family discipline for specific Bible study and reading of Christian novels, such as *The Chronicles of Narnia* by C. S. Lewis.

Our children were typical teenagers and our prayer throughout those years was for each of them to experience a total surrender to God's will for their lives. We knew this could occur only by their act of total consecration and the Spirit of God cleansing their hearts of self-interest — the same thing faced by every believer at a crisis point for total surrender.

Every child possesses self-centered attitudes that are amplified in the teen years and ours were no exception. One example in our household was Danielle when she was in seventh grade. An attitude of stubbornness began to manifest itself in her conversation and actions, and Loretta decided to take "the direct approach." She required Danielle to get up early in the morning before school and meet with her on the couch for prayer and study time together. As you can imagine, this did not please Danielle, and the first few days she showed her displeasure by sitting on one end of the couch with Loretta on the other. Slowly, however, Danielle inched her way toward her mom until they were beside one another in prayer. A definite change in Danielle became evident and she was empowered by the Lord to live a holy life for Him.

Our sons' discipleship included the "Young Timothy" studies we had as father and sons with other fathers and sons on a weekly basis. If a son was in a home without a father, we found an adopted spiritual father among our men in the church to join in the studies.

What molds children into disciples of Christ is the consistency of what they *observe being lived out* in the home aligning with what they are being taught. We had established our supper hour as our "regroup time" as a family before the heavy schedules started in the evening. One evening Loretta was serving the meal and in our conversation I became very short with her. Our children's faces reflected shock and confusion when they heard my disrespectful words to their mother. I immediately apologized to Loretta and asked for her forgiveness. I included the children in my apology, explaining to them that my words and attitudes toward their mother were not Christlike. It was a learning point in the application of the truth and a biblical worldview for our children.

When cancer attacked Loretta's body, it attacked our ministry as well. However, it attacked the wrong woman, the wrong family, and the wrong local church.

The result was a battle that for twenty-one years glorified God and His faithfulness, astounded the medical professionals, and gave witness for Jesus Christ: truly, **there is no other name but Jesus to call upon for salvation and healing.**

We often stated that we never would have volunteered for this journey, battling cancer, but we would not trade the benefits of what we jointly experienced and how God used it for His purposes.

Ed and Loretta Williamson

CHAPTER 4

AN UNEXPECTED DIAGNOSIS

The night before a scheduled hysterectomy in May of 1992, Loretta discovered a lump in her breast. She had been enjoying good health and was anticipating a routine recovery after the surgery. The lump concerned her, of course, so she mentioned it to her surgeon the next morning. "Well, we can't do two surgeries at the same time," he told her, "so let's talk about the lump on your post-op visit. We'll take a look at things then."

Loretta tolerated the hysterectomy well and even before her post-op visit, she got back into the swing of things. She was the administrator of the church's Christian school and with only two weeks until it was due to open, duties were pressing in on her. There were parents of prospective students to interview and, as happened every year, new children would be enrolling. This required a lot of energy and endurance. Uncharacteristically, Loretta began to tire quickly and experience shortness of breath and tightness in her chest. Her doctor had indicated that she could expect to recover from the surgery quite rapidly, but that just wasn't happening.

One night in particular, Loretta rushed home from work, got her family fed and retired early. She was so discouraged that she didn't even pray or read her Bible. She just fell into bed and went right to sleep. She later remarked that it is okay to feel discouragement, but it is not okay to remain discouraged and to blame it on God.

Even though Loretta felt downcast, she knew that she was in right standing with God and she took comfort from His Word. Psalm 18:21 states, *"For I have kept the ways of the Lord; I have not done evil by turning from my God."*

Loretta stirred as she heard me come to bed about 2:00 A.M. I had stayed up late to prepare for a funeral, as well as a wedding, the following day. Knowing I must be exhausted, she didn't say anything to me but as soon as I was breathing rhythmically and she knew I was sound asleep, she began to pray for me. She thanked the Lord for bringing us together and at some point she began to very quietly sing the song entitled, *No Other Name.* She wasn't in the habit of singing in bed; in fact, she didn't think she had a particularly good singing voice, but that didn't keep her from expressing herself in song. "No other name but the name of Jesus." Such beautiful words — and she thought she sounded so good that she softly sang again. As she did so, she entered into the presence of the Lord in genuine worship and felt His presence in a way she had never before experienced. It seemed her worship invited His tangible presence.

Since I was sound asleep, Loretta knew the Lord had not entered the room to meet with me, but had come to her. As this generation would express it, "It was awesome!" She began to sense His incredible love for her to the degree that she felt she could tell Him her deepest desires. In fact, she felt that was what He wanted her to do. His presence was just overwhelming. She didn't hear an audible voice or feel a touch, but He was there.

"Loretta," the Lord spoke to her heart, "I love you and I want to minister to you. Tell Me anything you want and give Me all your burdens. I'll carry everything for you."

So Loretta began to tell Him about the shortness of breath she was experiencing. "Lord, You know that I can't even take a deep breath because I feel so winded all the time. If You would just take care of that for me I'd so appreciate it."

She had taught kindergarten and was accustomed to doing a lot of motions with the children. One of their favorite stories was about the crippled man who was healed and began running and leaping and praising God. Of course, those motions were vigorous and she had been experiencing constrictions across her chest, reducing her lung capacity. That night she asked the Lord to relieve those symptoms, as well. Instantly, as though He cut the bands around her rib cage, she was able to take in deep, unrestricted breaths. She just lay there, taking time to inhale deeply and exhale freely, which encouraged her to ask the Lord for more.

"Lord, You know I must interview a prospective teacher for the third grade class and I really need discernment. This young woman is coming all the way from North Carolina and I want to do the right thing. You know that we don't need someone to just teach math and reading; we need someone who will love the kids and present the love of Christ to them."

She started talking to the Lord about the lump in her breast. "You know I am deeply concerned about the lump in my breast. It's starting to bother me and I'm always feeling to see if it's still there. I would sure appreciate it if You would just take care of it."

And then she added softly, "And, Jesus, I so desperately need your peace."

Finally, she started to pray for me. "Lord, I pray that Ed will experience a refreshing from the the Holy Spirit so he can do the wedding and the funeral tomorrow. He is such a good pastor and a wonderful husband and daddy and I thank You for him."

Starting to very quietly sing again, she drifted back to sleep with praises to God on her lips.

The next morning, Loretta could hardly wait to share with me about God's visitation and how she had felt so loved and cared for. She told me how she experienced total freedom to tell God her deepest desires, no matter how silly they might seem. Afterwards, I asked if she had asked the Lord for wisdom regarding our IRA. You see, we were preparing to send two of our children to Asbury College at the same time and we thought that if we cashed in our IRA and paid off the house, we might make the equivalent of our house payment to the college. We had been fervently praying for direction concerning that, but she told me that it never occurred to her to mention it to the Lord.

As a result of her time with God, Loretta no longer had shortness of breath. And in full confidence, she recommended to the school board that they hire the young lady from North Carolina for the third grade teaching position.

Two days later during her post-op visit, the surgeon examined the lump in her breast, and then sent her to a specialist in another building. Following that examination, she was sent for a mammogram. Technicians usually ask patients to wait before getting back into their street clothes so they can make sure they got a good image. In Loretta's case, a technician came to where she was waiting and told her, "You can get dressed now. Your doctor would like for you to go back to see him." Loretta explained that she already had an appointment scheduled for the following week, but the girl said, "No, he wants to see you now."

When Loretta sat down in the specialist's office, he asked her bluntly, "Where does your husband work?"

The serious tone of his question caused Loretta to catch her breath and anxiety gripped her. She hurriedly replied to the doctor and then called me; we made arrangements to meet in the parking lot as soon as I could get there. While she was waiting, she began singing, "No other name but the name of Jesus." She prayed and sang, prayed and sang, until I joined her.

I had been gearing up for a missions trip to Central Asia when I received Loretta's call saying the lump in her breast might be cancerous. I remember that the word cancer, when attached to my wife, felt like a slap across the face. Rushing to meet her, I wiped telltale signs of tears from my eyes and face as I held her in my arms and began praying with her before entering the doctor's office again.

Sitting together hand in hand, we heard the doctor say, "Loretta, I'm 98 percent certain that the lump is cancerous." His direct, matter-of-fact pronouncement was mind-numbing.

"I was able to get a report from your gynecologist and there was no hint of anything on your breast eleven months ago but there's something very prominent now. I'd like to put you under general anesthesia and do a biopsy."

Should the biopsy results be negative, I would be able to proceed with my trip to Central Asia. I felt certain that the lump would be benign and would not hinder my going on the trip, which I fully believed was God's will for me at the time. However, the biopsy report came back positive. As Loretta and I absorbed this blow, we had to decide whether to proceed with a mastectomy or a lumpectomy. Having a lumpectomy would require radiation as well as chemotherapy. We decided to go with the mastectomy, thinking it would be less taxing, and Loretta would be sufficiently healed for the opening of the school term.

Within a few days, Loretta was in surgery. I tried to shield her, as well as our children, from the impact of what was happening, but privately I was struggling with fear and anger. I felt uncertainty about facing the unknown without my Loretta, and while she was undergoing the mastectomy, I went to the prayer chapel in the hospital and wept.

My confidence was shaken because I had been so certain that God was going to heal my wife, and now she was losing her breast. I had assured her the night before that this assault on her femininity would do nothing to diminish my love for her or detract from her attractiveness to me. I expressed that my love was not based on physicality, but on her as a person and the wonderful wife and mother she was. I was to realize later that those words had to become incarnate, as the attack on her femininity had been successful.

I read the Psalms, and confessed my arrogance and error in "knowing God's will for her healing." However, I remember a profound assurance that cancer would not take her life and that our ministry together was not over. I simply could not envision my life without Loretta. Here are some of my thoughts concerning that period:

40

When I saw her in Recovery, I reassured her of my love and assured her that God was going to bring us through this together. Following her release from the hospital, I secured a few days at Canaan Valley Lodge in the mountains of West Virginia. The first time I saw her incision, I fought back the emotions that wanted to cry, "Unfair!" I held my "battle maiden" in my arms. If this was a spiritual attack against our ministry, I wondered why God was allowing Loretta to be the one to get beat up, cut upon, and subjected to such pain.

The Lord's earlier visit to Loretta fortified her for days of recovery at the hospital, which she liked to characterize as a spiritual retreat. The children and I were sustained and the Lord taught all of us how to go "through the valley of the shadow of death and fear not."

A particularly difficult experience occurred just two days after Loretta returned home. She was resting outside on the hammock and Danielle, our fifteen-year-old daughter, was assisting her in getting up. As she gently pulled Loretta out of the hammock, one of the drain tubes caught in the webbing of the hammock and the top flipped off, spraying both of them with blood. It splattered all over Danielle's face and Loretta began to cry. She was terribly upset to see her little girl having to deal with that when she should be having fun with friends. Danielle proceeded to clean up both of them, and then she creatively designed pockets to house the drain bottle, eliminating any future such occurrences. This clever design also enabled Loretta to attend church without revealing her medical paraphernalia.

Danielle recalls this experience, as well as her general emotional response to her mother's cancer.

I was only fifteen, and although the battle was fast and furious with Mom's mastectomy, at least I was able to jump in and do something: take care of the house, design the tank top for her chest tubes, and wash her hair.

I recall only two instances that were emotionally draining for me as I assisted with her care. The first was when I helped change her out of her hospital gown so she could come home following the mastectomy. I certainly knew that my mother had cancer and her right breast had been removed, but I had been able to remain somewhat detached from the situation. As I delicately untied her hospital gown, her incision was exposed and I remember wanting to cry — or even scream, "This is not fair! Look what cancer has done to my mother!" Not only had it literally eaten away part of her body, but also she was in so much pain that the simple task of getting dressed was taking much longer than usual.

Instead of allowing the tears that were suffocating my throat to escape, I swallowed with difficulty and gently guided Mom's arm through the sleeve of her blouse. At the time I thought the incision was what bothered me, but now I think it was more the role reversal as I cared for her. However, as difficult as it was, it was therapeutic for me to be able to do something to make life a little easier for my mother.

Draining her chest tubes was not problematic for me, although it was difficult to observe her suffering significant pain week after week. I recall washing her hair in the kitchen sink and afterward going into my bedroom, lying across my bed sobbing. How could I handle blood seeping from my mother's chest tube, but fall apart when washing her hair? It didn't make sense at the time, but I think that deep down I feared future treatments that could reduce her to a chronic, feeble state of health. Caring for Mom at these times was almost overwhelming, but overall I was glad to keep busy.

Mom was an excellent housekeeper and I did my best to ease her mind about maintaining an orderly house. Cancer leaves its victim and family feeling so desperate because there is seemingly so little to combat it. Caring for my mother seemed to be my only physical means of standing up to this disease.

Throughout this time our family learned how to really pray together. Weekly devotion times had been a tradition in our family and now these became times of battling cancer. Even mealtimes became opportunities to approach the throne of God. The constant prayers were certainly my stronger means of supporting Mom, but if the other tasks had been taken from me, I think I would have fallen apart much more easily.

As Mom's strength returned, I began to question God. "How could this have happened? Why my mother, who has dedicated her life to Christian ministry?" Just when we thought she was going to quickly recover from her hysterectomy, she was felled by this much more serious disease. I had been so sure that the biopsy would reveal a benign mass, or that they would find nothing. I had been so confident that the Lord would heal her. Did God not really mean what He promised?

The questions in my mind continued to grow, but I didn't relay them to anyone. I was ashamed of myself for even thinking such thoughts. After all, I had grown up in the church, and had a personal relationship with God. In fact, three years earlier I had given everything to the Lord: my future, my hopes, wherever He wanted me to go, whatever He wanted me to do. I just couldn't possibly understand why God would allow this to happen, so I kept silent and continued to pray for Mom's healing.

My mother's energy level increased, but the emotional changes she experienced from Tamoxifen (a medication that blocks estrogen and lowers the chance of a recurrence of cancer) were sometimes difficult to deal with. Something I said or did would somehow end up causing her to leave the room in tears. Before I recommitted my life to God at the age of twelve, I had become quite adept at being a smart aleck with my parents. But the Lord had changed me. I would never intentionally hurt my mother, and I wondered what I was doing wrong. Generally her strength and spirits were better than they had been in years, but these unpredictable changes made it seem that, in some ways, cancer had already taken her from us. Looking back, I recognize that this may have contributed to my hesitancy to completely trust the Lord with my mother's life.

As my distrust of my Savior grew, fear became my biggest enemy. Dreams of Mom dying plagued my sleep. Once I even dreamed that I had been asked to identify her body at the hospital. There she lay, completely naked, with her head bald and her body withered to almost nothing. I jolted awake with a sensation of falling.

Instead of feeling relief that it was just a dream, I was overwhelmed by a sense of darkness and evil, so much so that I was unable to speak. It felt like the air had been sucked out of my room and I couldn't breathe. There seemed to be a shadow at the foot of my bed, glaring down at me, crouching as if ready to pounce. I could only think the name of Jesus, unable to even move my lips. Slowly I was able to speak and I asked the Lord for His peace and protection. As suddenly as the image appeared, it was gone. Was it all part of a horrible dream? I don't know. I had always been skeptical of such stories, but one thing I know for certain, the fear I felt was almost tangible.

In the coming days, people's focus somehow seemed to switch from Mom to me. Friends at church would ask if I had been on a diet, and I started trying to wear baggier clothes to avoid being asked that so often. I had not intentionally lost weight, but after getting on the scales at Mom's promptings, I saw that I had lost nearly twenty pounds.

My dad had asked me to come up for prayer at the Sunday evening services, and while I couldn't say why, I avoided doing so for several weeks. I had been battling fear, and at some point the object of my fears changed. I was still fearful of losing Mom, but now I was afraid that I would be the next one to die. Not only was I terrified at the thought of cancer eating away at my body, but I was utterly ashamed that I harbored such fears. Here was my mother, the perfect example of a godly wife and mother, battling cancer and I had managed to turn the focus back to me.

Finally one Sunday evening my dad looked directly at me and, pointing, he beckoned me to the front of the church. Previously I had rationalized my not going forward as being because so many others in the church needed to talk and pray with him. However, I knew that I was afraid he would discover my selfishness at being fearful of being diagnosed with cancer, instead of focusing on my mother's continued healing.

As Dad laid hands on me and anointed me with oil, Mom and the church family gathered around me with their arms outstretched. Almost instantly my dad began to pray against the fear that had been plaguing my life for several months. A warmth started at my head and gently flowed down my entire body. I have never felt so loved and protected — and the fear was gone. Whenever the fear attempted to return, I gave it to the Lord and He continued to guide me in His peace, surrounded by His presence.

Nathan, our youngest child, was a "mama's boy" and unabashedly admitted it. Although he was only thirteen when Loretta was first diagnosed with breast cancer, he remembers his reaction well:

I cried and tried to understand why God would allow something like this to happen to Mom. My first thoughts were fairly simple, and mainly self-oriented. What would I do without Mom? If she died, then she would never get to see me grow up and graduate from high school or college. And she would never get to meet my future family here on earth. I think my greatest fear was just not having her in my life anymore. I simply couldn't imagine life without her. I don't take change well, in general; in fact, I remember once becoming quite upset over breaking a bowl that had been in the family since before I was born.

Then, my thoughts turned to Dad. What would he do without Mom? Would he marry someone else? I hoped that no one would ever take Mom's place in Dad's life if she went to heaven first. As I reflect now, I realize I didn't really know how to handle the situation. I had never experienced a close death, and now I was facing it square on. I prayed about it and I knew that God was in control.

At that point, I chose not to dwell on it or think about it anymore. I'm sure part of that was just immaturity. After all, I was still dependent on my parents for guidance and protection. I took my cues from them and since they were obviously trusting God, so did I. In fact, I was playing Nintendo Game Boy *in the hospital lounge while the doctors were performing Mom's mastectomy. It wasn't that I didn't care, I just didn't have the life experience to fully grasp the seriousness of our circumstances, and the game acted as an emotional detachment. Yet, I couldn't avoid seeing my dad focused in prayer and deep concentration, obviously heart-torn, but hopeful that God would bring her through. And He did!*

Ed and Loretta Williamson

CHAPTER 5

GROWING THROUGH TRIALS

Loretta badly wanted to attend church that first Sunday following her mastectomy simply to attest to the faithfulness of God. The wife of the assistant pastor graciously loaned her a casual suit with a loose jacket to cover all her "gear." Someone remarked that she looked radiant and she attributed that to the glow of the glory of the Lord.

The recovery in Loretta's right arm muscles was expedited through her writing on the chalkboard of her classroom, as well as raising it in praise to God . . . even when it hurt. The oncologist encouraged a series of chemotherapy treatments for extra assurance, but after much prayer, she declined. She began taking Tamoxifen, the standard protocol for an estrogen-fed cancer like hers. However, it presented its own problems. It is programmed to kill any estrogen in the body, causing immediate menopause with all its uncomfortable symptoms, including mood swings.

Our family pulled together and grew spiritually as a result of this trial, as did our church family. We did, in fact, call it all joy. In addition, the afterglow from Loretta's nocturnal visit with the Lord never left her.

In December 1993, Loretta's youngest sibling, George, died suddenly and traumatically and the effects of his death reverberated throughout the family. Loretta comforted the family with the possibility that the Lord had saved him before his death. Denise was inconsolable but during this time she and Loretta began to talk again after many years of estrangement. Grief over George's death had softened both their hearts and their relationship slowly grew and deepened.

Life gradually returned to normal in our household as we settled into long-established routines. Loretta gained strength and resumed many of her responsibilities and ministry duties, which was where she found such joy.

In February 1995, Loretta carpooled with some other women to Asbury College to visit our children, Ben and Danielle, and take them "care packages," as mothers love to do. Loretta so dearly enjoyed hearing Danielle play the piano, so they went to one of the campus practice rooms for an impromptu concert. It was while sitting there listening that Loretta began to feel chilled, and flu-like symptoms began to develop.

After her return home, for the next few weeks she ran a low-grade fever and experienced such pain in her ribs that when she coughed or sneezed she had to hold her sides to cushion the blow. No antibiotic sufficiently remedied the infection, so in April the doctor tried a round of medication designed for severe arthritis. That seemed to help for a while, but it only masked the pain.

Danielle recalls it this way:

> *I was a freshman at Asbury College and Mom had been doing quite well; despite some Tamoxifen-induced episodes, she was able to visit Ben and me for the weekend. As we walked around the campus, friends of mine would walk up to Mom and me and ask, "Now, which one of you is Danielle again?" We had a lot of fun together, and she seemed to feel quite well except for a cough that had developed, which hurt her ribs. I bundled her up in one of my sweatshirts, and then I played the piano for her. "How great to have a mother who is truly my best friend," I thought as I was playing. Later that year when I went home, I found out that Mom was going to have a bone scan, as the persistent chest pain that started that weekend had never gone away.*

Finally, in May, on the way home from a short trip to Boston, Loretta experienced extreme pain, and fear struck her heart. "Oh, oh," she thought, "I'm in trouble again." We called the doctor that night and he told her, "Loretta, we've got to get a bone scan because we must be sure the cancer hasn't returned."

Loretta had the scan performed the next day and then went on to school, thinking it might be a week or so before they heard the results. Ben and Danielle were in town from college and Nathan had been picked up from school, so we were all together at home when Loretta approached the back door after work. Glancing inside, she saw the look on my face and cried out, "What's wrong?" She thought I must have received bad news about a family member because I could hardly speak through my tears.

All I could say was, "Jeff," (my brother's name) so Loretta assumed that something had happened to him. Then she caught a glimpse of the children in the other room crying.

"What's wrong with Jeff? What happened?"

I finally composed myself enough to answer her.

"No, it's not my brother. Dr. Jeff called to say that you have cancer in your rib cage. It affects two ribs on one side and one on the other and they don't know if it has spread to your organs. But there is definite metastasis."

Dr. Jeff was a member of our church as well as our trusted physician and friend. When Loretta heard the report she immediately received a spiritual adrenaline rush and felt a righteous anger toward this demonic disease. As she said, "God never intended disease to be in this world. That came as a result of sin and the Fall."

I was completely broken at that moment so Loretta called the children into the room. We all gathered together and held hands in a circle of prayer.

"Let's just bring this to the Lord," Loretta said. "Let's take authority over this and believe God for a miracle."

Loretta had never been strong like that, so God's grace was beginning to work. God saw Loretta in her weakness and helped her become strong. She was especially burdened for our children, who felt forsaken by God with this devastating news. She and I joined in prayer that night that the Lord would fill the children with hope and peace. Danielle and Ben were having an especially hard time, perhaps because they were older and had to be away from home.

Nathan has expressed that he was always impressed with how

Loretta and I worked together in a "give and take" partnership over the years. When one of us seemed broken and weak, the other was fortified and carried the load until we regained our footing. That day our family's circle of prayer was a perfect example of this.

Nathan's fifteenth birthday was a few days later, so Ben and I went out and bought him a new stereo. We gave it to him a little early so that in the midst of such terrible grief, we were still able to celebrate.

Ben and Danielle went back to college and I often had to attend to church business in the evenings, so Nathan and Loretta were able to spend lots of time together. They were very similar in personality and the long talks they enjoyed seemed to help him through this confusing time. His journey of faith solidified, and he absorbed his mom's love and care as he shared his concerns about her life-threatening battle. They both appreciated the gift of time they had as they forged a deep bond.

Here are some of my recollections of what I felt and experienced emotionally after this, yet another dreaded diagnosis:

Loretta was the only one not badly shaken by this news. As I reflect on that moment, I believe it was one of those times that the Apostle Paul talks about as the gift of the Spirit ("effects of His power") being manifest in a believer's life. It was not a response of denial from Loretta, but one of assurance and anger toward this renewed cancer invasion of her body. This was one of my lowest points while dealing with this crisis.

What we discovered in the weeks following was that faith is not a rush of emotion, but rather the result of a calculated, planned saturation of the Word of God. His promises, through the comfort provided by peace from the Holy Spirit, grew our faith. As our knowledge grew, so did our faith. The prophet Hosea proclaimed, "My people die for lack of knowledge." The chorus I Will Sing of Your Love Forever *has a line that says, "And I will open up my heart and let the Healer set me free."*

We gained new insights and revisited several passages of Scripture in our battle for healing. We realized that divine healing is not in the heavenlies and suddenly falls down and heals the sick body. Healing begins from within the heart of the believer who is walking in fellowship with the Holy Spirit. Physical healing manifests through the body from within the spirit of the individual, not from outside into the person as in a sudden burst from heaven. The anointing with oil and the laying on of hands are acts of obedience to Scripture, agreeing that what God says is true. This outward act does not bring healing into an individual's body, but the prayer of faith agrees and joins with the diseased person's faith for the healing to be manifest within him.

Healing with the Word of God is what produces spiritual growth and increased faith in the heart of the individual. Our focus became single-minded toward Christ — concentrating on the Healer, Christ, and not on Loretta's healing. The focus was on what God's Word says about sickness, not the symptoms, pain, or medical diagnosis. We could sing, "I will sing of Your love forever," and in the midst of our pain, focus on Christ to open the door of faith in our hearts for the manifestations of His healing presence. The healing presence of Jesus in our worship services fed our hearts and soothed our emotions week to week.

Loretta began to read a book I had given to her entitled, *Healing: The Three Great Classics on Divine Healing* by Andrew Murray, A. J. Gordon, and A. B. Simpson. She was curious to know what these three highly respected men of faith had to say about divine healing. It was the beginning of a process of gathering all the evidence that she could find to encourage her in her belief that the Word of God is true.

One of the stories in the Bible that significantly bolstered her faith was the account of Abraham when God had promised him a son in his old age. The patriarch would not have believed if he had been looking for natural signs, as he was old and his wife was well past childbearing years. The Bible says that he considered not his own body, but the promises of God.

Loretta's entire family and a body of believers began to gather evidence to stir their hearts to believe the promises of God. She even prayed to consider that this might be God's timing to take her to be with Him. She figured that our children were older and all were serving the Lord. Yet, when she would contemplate my doing ministry alone, she felt that I really needed her at this time in the life of the church, which was experiencing some serious turbulence. Then, she considered whether this might just be a plot of Satan to discourage me and distract me from my work for God's kingdom. This became more firmly entrenched in her heart and she began to feel that we were to believe God for healing.

The Lord gave me a verse of Scripture that resonated with me:

> *"Though you search for your enemies, you will not find them. Those who wage war against you will be as nothing at all. For I am the Lord, your God, who takes hold of your*

right hand and says to you, Do not fear; I will help you"
(Isaiah 41:12).

I made posters of that verse and placed them around Loretta's classroom, as well as in our home. Students would slip Loretta notes with words of healing written on them. One morning she walked into her classroom to find it decorated with laminated posters, each with a promise of God. I was taking literally Proverbs 4:21: "Do not let my word out of your sight."

"What about the children, Lord?" Loretta was understandably concerned about them, and the Lord spoke this verse to her heart:

> *"All your sons will be taught by the Lord, and great will be your children's peace. In righteousness you will be established: tyranny will be far from you; you will have nothing to fear. Terror will be far removed; it will not come near you"* (Isaiah 54:13-14).

Those verses were exemplified in the lives of our three children as God met each of them with words of comfort and hope, always through His Word.

I relayed to Loretta that at one point I went up to Ben's room to check on him, only to find him on the floor, curled up in a fetal position, crying. Ben was a sophomore in college at that time and simply couldn't grasp that God had allowed cancer to reinvade his mother's body.

I continued to pray earnestly for the children that God would meet them and give them hope. God answered my prayers and met Ben in a supernatural manner early one morning. Loretta awoke that morning to find a letter from Ben under the door of our bedroom.

She immediately went downstairs to read his early morning "telegram."

Mom, It is about 1:33 A.M. I couldn't sleep so I went downstairs to get a drink and came back up and started reading the Word. I opened up immediately to Isaiah 43:1-2. Remember when you gave me this verse to put up in my room when I was in junior high school? You told me to put my name in for the word "you" and to hold on to the promises written in the verse. Well, now I think that the Lord has given me this verse to give back to you, so you can put your name in and stand on the promises.

> *But now, this is what the Lord says –*
> *He who created (Loretta), O Jacob*
> *He who formed (Loretta), O Israel*
> *Fear not, for I have redeemed (Loretta);*
> *I have summoned (Loretta) by my name;*
> *(She) is mine.*
> *When you pass through the waters, I will be with you;*
> *And when you pass through the rivers,*
> *They will not sweep over you.*
> *When you walk through the fire, you will not be burned;*
> *The flames will not set you ablaze.*

Mom, I am standing with you on those promises. We serve a God who is faithful to His Word and therefore we have nothing to fear. Dad always said in his sermons that God has taken away the dragon's teeth, so he can only gum us to death. This demon of cancer may look intimidating, but if we stand on God's promises he is all bark and no bite. Continue to be strong. The rivers will not wash over you and the fire will not burn you. Keep your eyes on Jesus and Him alone and He will pull you through. I have felt God reassuring me that we, as a family, are in His hands and under His protection. I love you and am continuing to stand on the victory that is ours in Christ Jesus.

Your son – Ben

Ben recalls that experience with these words:

I remember wanting to be strong for Mom and put on a brave face, hiding the fears that I felt. My desire was to be a help to her and the family, and I thought the best way to accomplish this was to grieve alone.

With this recurrence of cancer I kept asking God, "Why was this allowed to happen to my mom? Why us? She is and has been Your faithful servant, but where is Your faithfulness? Where is Your justice?" I remember the night that the Lord answered my questions. He was there in my room in such a real way, and I began to weep in His presence. I opened my Bible and read Isaiah 43:1-2. I remembered Mom giving me this scripture when she thought I was having a difficult time in junior high school (she was right, as usual). She had told me to insert my name into the scripture and stand on the promises given there.

I felt the Lord telling me that He was there, present and in control. The fear departed and I started rejoicing. I felt like Joshua when he met the commander of the armies of the Lord on his way to Jericho. The battle was now the Lord's, not mine. The armies of the Lord were there and I had no need to fear because He is the God who keeps all His promises to His faithful ones. I wrote a letter to Mom that night telling her about my visit from the Lord, and slipped it under her door.

Loretta stated that it is easy to rely on one's own strength and resources, and forget what is ours as adopted sons and daughters of our heavenly Father. When storms assail us, we feel helpless because we aren't accustomed to relying on the Lord and His promises. Sometimes we even feel abandoned by Him. Yet, it begs the question: Who really does the abandoning? She confessed that even after her first bout with cancer, she had failed to rely completely on the Lord. She felt that her prayerlessness had rendered her vulnerable to an attack of fear. But she was just as quick to give praise to her heavenly Father, who, through His divine mercy, comforted her in His arms and let her know that He was her covering, protection, and defender.

She recalled that in the Old Testament, God repeatedly protected and defended the widow, the fatherless, the weak, and the downtrodden. When we are powerless, He is our strength! She also considered that if God could speak words of life and hope to her through her twenty-year-old son at 1:33 in the morning, then she had nothing to fear. She came to understand that we truly were in God's hands and under His protection. Furthermore, she was confident that God's words are life to those who find them and health to a man's whole body.

We received the news that the cancer had returned on a Thursday, and we shared it with the teachers at school during staff meeting the next day. The administrator led the teachers in prayer as they laid hands on Loretta and that became a part of their daily prayer time after that.

The following Sunday I had to share it with our congregation; we wanted our church family to know so that they could do battle with us as they had many times before. I did the opening announcements, paused, and then said, "Loretta's bone scan indicated that the cancer is back." I broke down and wept and Loretta, overcome with compassion, went up on the platform and stood next to me.

"God spoke to my heart," Loretta began. "When He told that 'old man' Abraham that he and his 'old wife' were going to have a baby, Abraham considered not his body but rather the promises of God. Likewise, I am not to consider my body and these ribs and this cancer invasion, but rather the promises of God." She knew that His Word would be medicine to her bones. She was so confident in the Lord's ministering of this truth to her that she gained a supernatural hope that these scriptures applied to her situation.

In our first visit to Oncologist #1, the scan indicated hot spots on two ribs on Loretta's right side and one on her left, exactly where she was experiencing pain. The doctor described the recommended protocol: Loretta would be in isolation, as her immune system would be weakened, then her bone marrow would be removed and frozen. Her system would then be bombarded with heavy doses of chemotherapy.

The oncologist recommended a thoracic surgeon to do a biopsy of the ribs and Dr. Jeff said of him, "He is an excellent surgeon; I would let him operate on my own mother."

While the medical professionals were gathering their data, Loretta and I were gathering evidence from God's Word demonstrating that His healing power is relevant today.

One evening Loretta overheard Danielle scolding her younger brother Nathan because he indicated that it wouldn't be so bad if their mom died, as she would just go to heaven where we all hoped to go someday. Danielle was impatient with him, believing that he was just spouting platitudes that he hadn't processed. She was afraid he was in denial, avoiding the possibility that their mother might die.

Nathan remembers thinking that he and his brother and sister needed to remain strong for Loretta and me. His faith was solidly his own and he knew that he could rest in the hands of his heavenly Father. "In addition," he states, "I knew that Mom's and Dad's strength continued to carry over to me. My siblings and I helped around the house as much as we could, although we did everything with a sense of urgency. And we enjoyed each moment we had with Mom as if it were our last, even though we kept believing for God's healing."

On the day of surgery, a second oncologist, whose sons attended our church school, dropped by Loretta's room and offered to pray with her. This encouraged her and then later, when she awakened from anesthesia, the surgical nurse, who attended our church, greeted her with praises to God.

Loretta's lung had collapsed during surgery and she woke up with a chest tube in place and a seven-inch incision under her left breast. She had to be given morphine to help control excruciating pain. Her friend Cindy Rios, who was also battling breast cancer, dropped by for a visit and left behind a tape by John Hagee entitled, "The Healing Scriptures." God would later use the teachings on this tape to carry Loretta through some difficult days.

At one point during Loretta's hospital stay, a nurse inadvertently pressed hard against the incision site on her rib cage. The pain was so severe that she nearly passed out. The nurse quickly administered an injection of pain medication, but the pain persisted. On her way to have more x-rays, Loretta encountered Oncologist #2 again. She was crying and, of course, he asked what was happening. She told him about her painful experience and his response was less than sympathetic. He told her that he was reading a book about the early martyrs and encouraged her to consider what they must have suffered, adding that it might help to alleviate some of her distress. At the time she didn't find it very comforting.

Loretta began to feel so alone in the hospital! I was needed at church, the two older children had begun their summer jobs, and Nathan was still in school. She called me, hoping for some consolation. Unfortunately, I was tied up with work at church and couldn't get away but I had her friend Libby go to be with her. God had healed Libby of cervical cancer and she was happy to encourage Loretta. The next day Loretta received the good news that there was no evidence of cancer in her soft tissue.

Loretta was still hospitalized on Sunday and the entire church was praying for her. She acutely needed this prayer support because she had begun to inquire, "Lord, is it my time?" In her own words:

> *I know everyone has to die; in fact, we are all dying. So I was saying to the Lord, "I know that to live is Christ, to die is gain. And I am so comforted to know that my children all know You personally."*

> *But then I thought about Ed. "Oh, Ed needs me. We are a team in ministry and I have to stay here and be his teammate." When that reality hit me, it strongly motivated me and I proceeded to believe God for my healing.*

The Lord spoke directly to her heart through this verse in Psalm

118:17: *"I will not die but live, and will proclaim what the Lord has done."* She clung to those words, "I will not die."

Her hospital stay seemed unusually protracted for just a biopsy. She wanted to go home because there were things at school that concerned her. For instance, she would miss the kindergarten class graduation. Our daughter, Danielle, who is gifted in working with children, agreed to assist with coordinating that. It was a tall order for a college kid, but she did a wonderful job, according to her proud mom. Loretta came to realize that her class was in very capable hands and she could concentrate on getting better. In addition, Debbie, a friend and a nurse at the hospital, spent her free time praying with Loretta and encouraging her. Because of her position, Debbie was able to act as a medical liaison for the family. She went the extra mile and kept Loretta's two sisters apprised of her progress. They were both nurses and were concerned that Loretta was getting the best of care.

Finally Loretta was able to be released from the hospital and she was home alone when her lab report came in. Oncologist #1 personally called to say that he could hardly believe the results: NO CANCER.

"Loretta, I'm reading and rereading the pathology reports and looking at the slides. Everything says negative but I'm having a hard time believing it. I think we're going to need to do a few more tests. If the reports hold up, *then* I'll get excited."

Loretta told him that she had no difficulty believing the good report. Of course, she immediately phoned me. I was out shopping and when I heard the news I started singing a hymn of praise. I then called the two children at school and quoted this portion of Isaiah 41:12: *"Though you search for your enemies, you will not find them; those who wage war against you will be as nothing at all."*

Loretta had the assistant pastor contact Nathan with the news and asked him to quote the scripture to him, as well. The family was in one accord and praising God together.

Later that evening Loretta called Oncologist #2, who had offered to answer any questions she might have.

"Doctor, have you heard the good news?"

"Well, Loretta, I *want* to rejoice with you but I think there's a problem. I have seen the pathology reports and I believe there's been a mistake." Loretta was taken aback. He was a Christian doctor and she had hoped that he would be rejoicing with her.

"What are you saying, Doctor?"

"You have metastasis to your ribs. I know you do. So I'm not going to believe the reports until they are confirmed. I would really like for you to have another bone scan."

Loretta consented to the scan and later that week when this doctor called and said that the report was accurate, he added a jolting remark: "We have determined that the biopsy was done on the wrong rib! That's why nothing shows up."

After hearing these discouraging words, Loretta listened to "The Healing Scriptures" read by John Hagee all that evening so that doubts would not overcome her spirit.

The next day she made it to "Water Day" at the preschool and shared the doctors' doubts with the other teachers. That evening she worked on report cards and got psyched for the last half-day session of school and the closing program and picnic with the students and their parents.

A few days after the close of school, Loretta and I were once again waiting our turn to be seen by Oncologist #1. We really had to be prayed up when we waited for those appointments, as there were times it felt like death surrounded us and we were marked to be its next victim. It doesn't matter if you are young or old, male or female, death by cancer is no respecter of persons.

Finally Oncologist #1 met with us, stating that he had not expected the results. He had called on three radiologists to view the bone biopsy, as he wasn't used to receiving negative results on a bone scan for metastasized breast cancer. He requested that Loretta have one more bone scan to rule out the possibility that the wrong rib was again scanned. She was all too happy to comply because it would confirm what God had done.

Danielle went with her for the scan and the family continued to trust God and His Word.

Loretta called Oncologist #1 the following Monday to get the results of the scan and Linda, his nurse, stated that she would call for them. Loretta didn't hear anything from them so she called again on Wednesday to request that the report be sent to the thoracic surgeon's office in time for her appointment that afternoon. Linda assured Loretta that they would be there.

Loretta and I arrived early to the thoracic surgeon's office with a copy of her chest x-ray. As the resident examined and cleaned her incision, she asked him about the bone scan.

"Oh, that report is back."

"How does it look? Is everything fine?"

"Well, the scan was scheduled for rib #5 but they had requested rib #4." The resident said this all very matter-of-factly and neither Loretta nor I picked up on the import of his words.

The thoracic surgeon, who was usually a smiling, pleasant man, entered the room with a grim expression. His tone was very businesslike as he spoke to us. He stated that he had felt all of the ribs on one side and ordered a biopsy of the distorted one. He never indicated that the scan revealed any problems, but he did offer to scan the other side if we wanted to be sure. That seemed pointless since there was nothing to indicate a real need for it, so Loretta declined. She remarked that we were trusting God for a miracle.

As we left his office, Loretta remarked to me that she felt the staff was uncomfortable with us and were even withholding information. At this point she determined to speak with Oncologist #1 as soon as possible. Her anxiety level was rising and she feared that our miracle was in jeopardy.

The next day, she called the office of Oncologist #1 and told Linda that she had lots of questions for the doctor. Linda assured her that she would have him call her when he arrived in the office. When Loretta didn't receive a callback by late that afternoon, she called again only to learn that he had not come into his office that day.

Linda picked up on her anxiety and asked, "Would you like for me to read what the pathology report said?"

Of course, Loretta did so Linda continued, "Now there are four ribs and he cut a healthy rib. That's why the report is negative."

This indicated that the thoracic surgeon did, in fact, biopsy the wrong rib. Again, Loretta felt terribly alone and she broke down in tears. Why hadn't anyone told her? Were they worried about a lawsuit? She had suffered a collapsed lung and unspeakable pain with nothing to show for it. Nothing!

I was engaged in church work and the children were at summer jobs, so out of desperation Loretta attempted to reach one of the doctors. She reached his wife and found out that he was in Chicago for the weekend. In her fear, anger and frustration, Loretta felt free to share with the doctor's wife and, regrettably, she began to understand why people sue doctors. While Loretta conceded that mistakes are unavoidable, skirting directness and honesty with patients actively seeking answers is not.

Actually, several persons told Loretta and me that we had a powerful case against the hospital and the surgeons for operating on the wrong rib. But I responded, "How can we sue them when we asked God to guide the hands of the surgeon?" Loretta was in complete agreement but we did get one thing out of it. The hospital dismissed our bill for the surgery.

Dr. Jeff provided the first bit of encouragement by stating that he would meet with the thoracic surgeon and Oncologist #1. Bone scans can turn out to be false positives and he advised Loretta to just sit tight. He was encouraged by the fact that her pain had diminished.

It was almost time for church camp to begin and I desperately wanted Loretta to accompany me so she could rest and aid her recovery. I feared that if she stayed home alone, she might get depressed.

That same day, Loretta received a phone call from Harold Thompson, our denomination's District Superintendent, stating that although the doctors may have made a mistake, that didn't change what God was going to do. He encouraged her to continue to believe that God was working and that His will wasn't contingent on what man does.

She felt assured that the Lord really used Pastor Harold that day, as she couldn't convince herself that everything was going to be fine.

God honors our trust and expectation of Him to work and move, even in the toughest of situations. Hebrews 10:23 says, *"Let us hold unswervingly to the hope we profess, for He who promised is faithful."* Verses 38-39 were a further reminder to her:

> *"But my righteous one will live by faith. And I take no pleasure in the one who shrinks back. But we do not belong to those who shrink back and are destroyed but to those who have faith and are saved."*

Later that day during her devotions, Loretta came across Psalm 25:3: *"No one whose hope is in you shall ever be put to shame."* She decided not to dwell on bone scans or botched biopsies; her hope would be in the Lord. She was even further blessed to find this assurance in Psalm 112:7: *"He will have no fear of bad news; for his heart is steadfast, trusting in the Lord."* She praised the Lord for meeting her once again through His powerful, awesome Word; and once again she was able to focus on His truth, not on her circumstances.

Shortly after this, Denise, Loretta's younger sister, came to visit. Denise, who has a PhD in health policy from Brandeis University, could not believe that a competent surgeon would cut the wrong rib. Loretta tried to convince her that her doctors were totally competent and considered among the best in their field. But the fact that the thoracic surgeon had gone with the wrong rib upset her.

Denise allowed Loretta to talk about Jesus more than she usually had, as their relationship had strengthened. They had a terrific time together and Denise helped Loretta with her annual plantings in the front of the house. The entire family was a witness to the peace that Jesus had instilled in us, including our children, Ben, Danielle and Nathan.

Loretta and I were departing for camp the same day that Denise was catching a plane to return home. Ben, who was working two summer jobs, was drafted to take her to the airport. He hoped to be able to witness to his aunt, now that he was twenty years old and could communicate his faith cogently. The other family members were just hoping he would not get so distracted by his efforts to share his faith clearly that he would miss his airport exit.

I was the guest camp speaker, and Loretta was to be available for ministry and counseling with the girls on an as-needed basis. Otherwise, she had no particular assignment, and she could get some needed rest. She was not going to neglect being active for the Lord just because her healing wasn't complete. We were pressing on by faith and the Lord was blessing our efforts. We were there as a team, each expecting the Lord to work and use us, trusting Him to take care of the physical body as we did business with the spiritual man.

Once we were settled in, the camp director asked Loretta if she could fill in for a pastor's wife who had become ill. Her duties would entail teaching a daily forty-five-minute seminar to a group of high school students. The topic was "The Anvil" and Loretta was challenged by the subject matter. She realized that the director had placed a lot of confidence in her ability, so she accepted the assignment but, by her own admission, she didn't do so joyfully. Loretta was not a fly-by-the-seat-of-your-pants type of person. She didn't want to look foolish in front of others, and this particular assignment didn't allow much preparation time. I gently reminded her that the Lord was her helper.

As it turned out, that teaching on the anvil was just what Loretta needed, perhaps more than the students. God ministered His truths to her both in the classes and in the evening services. Many young people gave their lives over to the lordship of Jesus Christ, renouncing those things that had held them back. In spite of enjoying refreshing times of teaching, however, she tired easily and had to rest each afternoon. That week turned out to be one of the best of her life and healing continued to take place in her body.

Loretta had not brought her Tamoxifen to the camp with her because she didn't want to experience the awful mood swings the drug induced and, anyway, she was only continuing it to appease her mom, who regularly asked if she was taking it. It was a drug with uncomfortable side effects: hot flashes, night sweats, mood swings, sexual disinterest and general discomfort. Even with all of its unpleasantness, she had reluctantly continued to take it off and on for almost three years.

When we returned home from camp, Loretta's sister Bernadette and three of her five children came from Massachusetts to visit. She later told Loretta that she had come to tell her good-bye. She, like Denise, is a nurse who felt that Loretta's diagnosis implied a poor prognosis because the cancer had metastasized to the bones. While Denise had planted flowers, Bernadette painted the front porch. Loretta and I had been finishing up our latest home improvement project when she was felled by cancer and we welcomed the help. Bern would get up early each morning and start painting before the heat became unbearable.

Because the sisters lived almost twelve hours from us, their visits were rare. Loretta and I made the trip to Massachusetts almost every year to visit her mom and dad and were able to see her sisters then. Difficulties in Bern's life and marriage had caused her to drift from the Lord and Loretta had hopes that they would have time to talk since Bern was so tender toward her. Bernadette's daughter Sarah is Danielle's age, and she requested that the family sing hymns and choruses in the evenings. Danielle played the piano and everyone sang and had worship. It was such a joyous visit.

Bernadette recognized changes in Loretta's personality that she thought were induced by Tamoxifen. She suggested that she accompany Loretta to the West Virginia University medical library to check it out. They discovered that Loretta had suffered the worst possible side effects. The conclusion of one study indicated that the benefits of Tamoxifen were greatest between the first and second year of usage and no significant differences were noted in the number of contralateral cancers among patients receiving two or five years of Tamoxifen.

Loretta decided to discontinue its use and she was grateful to the Lord for using her sister as a catalyst for doing what she felt He had given her permission to do. Above all, she didn't want her family blaming God for what they might perceive as an overly optimistic faith should she die. She felt God's Word was saying that she was being healed, while her physicians were saying that she was in denial.

Two more big events were coming up: our denominational northern junior camp in Doddridge County Camp, WV, and a trip to Disney World as guests of Loretta's brother, Armand. Junior camp went well, but the weather was extremely hot. Over one hundred campers attended and there were terrific counselors to work with them. Loretta had not been given any particular assignment and the kids and I were smiling from ear to ear when she intervened during a session of aerobics to Christian music. That had been her assignment in the past and it was her forte. When the participants struggled to remember the motions and missed the best part, she jumped in and led the way. She continued to do this twice daily and loved it! We all thought, "Is Mom being healed?"

We returned home from junior camp and prepared for our departure to Disney World in Orlando, Florida. Loretta found herself entertaining thoughts about the memories they would be building and how they would be special to the kids and me after she was gone. She resolved that her times were in God's hands and she was going to have a good time making those memories. Her good time was marred, however, when she developed a stiff neck and bone pain during the trip. Always looming in her thoughts was the idea that the bone cancer was spreading and that she should be seeking treatment. Yet, she continued to pray, "Lord, I believe. Help my unbelief."

In spite of Loretta's discomfort, that vacation turned out to be one of total relaxation. She spent time sharing a huge hammock with her brother as they reminisced about their lives before they found the Lord. She had witnessed to Armand shortly after her own conversion when he was home on leave from the Air Force. He had listened and resolved to become a better Roman Catholic. Bernadette and Loretta told him they would pray that God would bring someone in his path who would echo their message.

Armand testified fourteen years later that everywhere he went, including Japan and Thailand, someone was there who shared the gospel with him. He finally wore down and decided that God must really love him if He would chase him around the world. He is now a faithful disciple of Jesus Christ and a soul winner. He and his wife are serving the Lord in Tampa, Florida.

When the family returned from our week with Armand and Irma, another physician from our church called us. She said the doctors felt Loretta was in denial and that she should be following up with them regarding the unresolved bone scan. By this time, Loretta was sufficiently healed from the biopsy and was off the Tamoxifen. She felt little to no pain where her ribs were diseased, and coughing and sneezing were no longer excruciating experiences. Several more Christian friends called to say that the Lord had burdened them to pray for her and they were doing so. One lady even stated that she was doing battle in prayer for her.

On August 1, as we were waiting to see Oncologist #1 after two months of silence, Oncologist #2 came by to talk to us. He stated his concern for Loretta and the predicament she was in. She asked him if the doctors were certain about their cancer diagnosis. She further relayed to him how well she felt and that she and I felt the Lord was healing her.

"Loretta, I believe in prayer," he said. "My mother was diagnosed with advanced lymphoma and went through the usual course of chemotherapy. The treatments made her extremely ill and rather than watch her suffer, we decided just to put her in God's hands."

When he said that, Loretta realized that people do all they can do and *then* turn it over to God. "Why do we just about kill someone and get no results and then we put it in God's hands?" At that moment, she and I decided to turn our situation completely over to God. He had given us many reasons to believe Him trustworthy.

"Doctor, what would you do if your wife were in my situation?"

He responded, "I would advise her to have the procedure and then we would pray about it."

Loretta and I told him that we were still gathering evidence and asked him to keep us in prayer. Loretta committed to trusting God for her miracle and kept questioning why people tend to make Him their last resort.

When Oncologist #1 spoke with us, he stated that he understood our decision not to want another bone biopsy.

"I'm so sorry about what happened. The thoracic surgeon even called me during surgery and told me he knew that it wasn't the right rib but it looked like the best specimen. So he didn't do this haphazardly — it wasn't a mistake. He strongly felt that he observed disease in the other rib as well."

Loretta was not in rebellion against the doctors. However, though not planning to sue, she and I were determined not to pay any amount over what the insurance would cover. It was, after all, an unwarranted procedure.

Oncologist #1 advised us to keep a record of everything that had gone on and asked if Loretta would consent to another bone scan to check for further spread of the disease. She told him how well she felt off the Tamoxifen and then shared the research she and her sister had done on that drug study. He agreed that was a viable choice for her, especially in light of her uncomfortable side effects.

Loretta highly respected Oncologist #1 for allowing her to make choices about her treatment without his feeling threatened. As she waited for his nurse to give her a date for the bone scan, she told the doctor that we were still trusting God to heal her, a healing to which all the doctors would bear testimony.

CHAPTER 6

PROBLEMS IN MANY FORMS

In August, my mom called telling us that my dad had been in a head-on collision. He was being transferred from their local Parkersburg hospital to a heart specialist in Morgantown to determine if he had suffered a heart attack. Thanks to his air bag, he was going to survive the accident, and the other driver escaped unharmed. It was evident that my dad was in the wrong lane, but why he had veered there was unclear. After many tests, it was determined that his heart had caused him to lose consciousness and he would be fitted with a pacemaker.

With grateful hearts, Loretta and I were able to spend time with him in the hospital as he convalesced. One day I was called away to take a phone call and when I returned to the hospital room Loretta could see that I was quite upset. I took her out into the hall and had to tell her that five of our teachers had decided not to sign their contracts for the upcoming school year. We had lost our previous administrator mid-year and so the associate pastor, who was experienced in Christian schools, had reluctantly completed the year. He was unhappy in this position, however, as he had inherited some unresolved conflicts that had to be dealt with. Some of his decisions were seriously questioned and this brought about a mass resignation of teachers.

Loretta instantly felt that this situation spelled the death of our school and she wanted to get right to work calling the parents so they could enroll their children elsewhere. My response was just the opposite: Our school would open on time! My reaction angered Loretta, as she felt I was not fully grasping the task that lay ahead of us.

"Ed, how can we possibly fill the five vacancies with Christians who are called and certified to do the job? Do you know how long this process will take?"

"Yes, I understand the enormity of the job. But I feel that this whole situation is the work of Satan adding to the death all around us here in this hospital. My dad has just had a close brush with death; you have the curse of death in your body; and now here is the sentence of death to the Christian school. Don't you sense the significance of all this?"

It was apparent to me that we were in a battle and we should not run, but rely on the Lord to rescue us. I immediately solicited the prayers of the parents, and their response was overwhelming. Only one family withdrew their children from the school. After meeting with the local church Board of Stewards, one of the five teachers decided to stay. The board also decided to eliminate the high school program and concentrate its energies and resources on pre-K through eighth grade.

The news that the school would open with a full complement of teachers was met with tremendous relief. The associate pastor declined the offer to take the position of administrator so I offered to fill the position until a replacement could be found. Soon after, the associate pastor resigned, taking approximately seventy members with him to begin a new church. Some of those leaving had been won to Christ through my ministry.

This proved to be the saddest time in our ministry! It was so painful that it became the only time Loretta and I considered leaving the ministry altogether. It was a near-mortal wound for me, although I acknowledge some complicity in what led up to that point.

School opened and Loretta and I offered praise to the Lord for His incredible feats. Yet, I was now head pastor of a wounded and bleeding church family and faced with some families who were divided and struggling to choose whom to follow. Sheep know the scent of their shepherd and will follow him, but it appeared these sheep had lost the scent of the shepherd. I was also the headmaster of the school and Loretta assisted where she could. In addition, the youth group had been in a slow decline. Loretta and I wondered if anything else could go wrong.

During the turbulence of the church split, our children did not know what was being said about Loretta and me and they didn't understand why people were leaving. Nathan was experiencing sudden, painful loss, as friends he had grown up with in the church were gone overnight. It was a bewildering time for all of us, but especially for a high schooler. Loretta and I trusted the Lord to keep us steady and Nathan told us later that our faith kept him strong in the midst of the upheaval.

As a result of the church problems, Nathan, now in the eleventh grade, started attending public school for the first time. Loretta and I took time to help him start a prayer group in our kitchen before school with the few friends he still had. It was a busy, sometimes chaotic, time as we faced cancer again, ran the school, pastored the church, and concentrated on the youth group.

Within a week of all the drama surrounding the church, Loretta realized that it was time for her scheduled bone scan. We had been too busy to think about it and since she wasn't in pain, it was easy to forget. However, it was on the calendar and so she went in on a Friday morning, reporting back to school for the afternoon session.

Loretta and I realized that we had a very high hill to climb, but we knew the Lord would be with us on the ascent. Looking back at how He had shown Himself faithful and powerful many times in the past increased our courage. Loretta recalled looking at me and realizing how proud she was to be my wife. But it was hard, no doubt about it.

At one point, when Sunday after Sunday we still weren't sure what accounted for some absences, Loretta said to me, "How many more have to leave before you realize it's over and God needs to put someone else in our place?"

"If I thought leaving Covenant would rescue it, then I would turn in my notice immediately. The only reason I'm staying is because I so deeply love the people. I feel that if I leave the church in such a fragile state, it will die." And that was unthinkable to me.

In order to get clear confirmation, Loretta and I invited the key leaders and their spouses to our home to examine the matter. We were ready to offer our resignation if they felt it would be best for the church. However, the unanimous voice of the leaders was that we should stay and they pledged to stand with their pastors. The gathering was concluded with the reading of Isaiah 61:3, the verse God had given to Loretta and me when the church was planted: God will raise up *oaks of righteousness, a planting of the Lord* around the ministry for protection, enabling it to withstand the storms that would surely arrive.

Loretta never again asked me to leave, but resolved to stand beside me and together we would be agents of God to bring healing to the church.

All of this had left our daughter, Danielle, very shaken. Cancer affects the entire family, each member in his or her own way. Danielle had this to say following Loretta's second cancer diagnosis, and the troubles within the church we pastored.

> *I was home from school for only four days when we received the call from Dr. Jeff. I overheard my dad talking with him on the phone, and I recall the way that his usually confident voice cracked as his muffled words escaped between quick gasps for air.*
>
> *I ran to my room. This could not be happening again. Not again! Knowing what was coming before anyone told me, I hid in my room. I tried to convince myself that I was wrong, that I just had a flair for the melodramatic. I willed myself to believe that I had misinterpreted the phone conversation, and I went back downstairs.*
>
> *As soon as I saw my dad's face, I wanted to run back to my room and slam the door. Do not say it! I wanted to scream, and then a sudden realization hit me. This is it. She is going to die. I knew it because I had never seen my dad look the way he did at that moment. The hopelessness*

in his deep-set eyes poured out over his face. Suddenly I felt a sharp pain in my hands. Looking down, I realized that my fists must have been clenched for several minutes, as my knuckles were white. While my dad's response seemed to be hopelessness, mine was anger.

My mom arrived home and my brothers and I hung back as my dad attempted to tell her the news. I was afraid to face her. What would her reaction be? Our faithful God had already prepared her for the battle when we were at our weakest. She simply held my dad and reassured him that God was still in control. We came together for a group hug and cried together.

In the coming weeks, my fear of losing my mother grew, as well as my fear of losing my faith in God. I was totally confident, prior to her mastectomy, that my mom would be found to be cancer free. When the news came back that she had cancer, I felt that the wind was literally knocked out of me. Realizing that God can work through medicine, I eventually came to see that the mastectomy was one of God's means of healing my mom. I certainly had fear during that first battle with cancer, but the second bout proved to be a much fiercer battle. It had completely blindsided me and I began to realize that my faith wasn't as strong as I thought. "If everything I believed was really true, why did the cancer come back?" I reasoned.

My struggle became apparent to my parents after the botched biopsy of her rib. Mom was rejoicing in the negative scan results, and I remained relatively silent. During one conversation, with a raised voice, Mom inquired of me, "Why aren't you excited about this?" While I didn't want to *tell her the whole truth and, being fearful that she would see through me if I totally dodged the question, I told her that I wanted to be absolutely sure of the results. I was so fearful that if I truly believed God had again healed my mom, and it turned out He hadn't, then that would be a fatal blow to my faith in Him. I hated myself for thinking that and I knew that if my mom knew what I was really thinking, it would be more devastating to her than the cancer that was in her body.*

The news of the mistaken rib brought me some relief that I hadn't placed all my hope in a clear bone scan. However, I was clearly choosing to take control of my emotions instead of simply trusting the Lord. I found that I didn't want to leave my mom's side. Perhaps in some way I was beginning the process of saying good-bye to her. We had frequent long talks and we both cried about the possibility that she wouldn't be there to attend my wedding some day. Through all of this, I never stopped praying for her healing. I had given my life to God when I was twelve years old, never imagining that I would have to put my mother's life into His hands just three years later.

When I received word at college about the turmoil in the church family, I battled anger as well as bitterness. On top of everything else, this was a near deathblow to my faith. I simply couldn't understand how Christians, the same ones who had taught me Bible verses in Sunday school and given me animal crackers in VBS, could be acting as they were. Many had vacationed with us; their children were my friends; my dad had answered their nocturnal calls for prayer when their children were having surgery;

and my parents had spent hours counseling them through both physical and spiritual struggles. How could they turn against my parents, especially now, when they were in the greatest battle of their lives? Yet, my parents continued to seek and trust the Lord. Never once did they question the sovereignty of God. They continued to place their hope in God, and brought others to surround them and do battle in prayer. This provided a great example of God's faithfulness even in the midst of unimaginable pain.

It was after my return to college that I came to a place of total abandonment before God. I was completely honest with Him. While I was no longer able to provide any physical support for my mom, I entrusted her to His care and keeping. I told God that if He took her home to be with Him, I would continue to serve Him with my whole being. My life (and my mother's life) were totally His. As I released my anger and fears to Him, the Lord replaced them with His love and peace. Just as He did for my parents, God placed people of strong faith around me to help sustain me during this period.

I would never have chosen this path for my family, but the blessings are numerous: a tightly-knit family that supports each other in the Lord; lasting friendships with fellow Christians; a new sense of awe and wonder at God's power and grace; and the opportunity to share with others so that they may come to know God through Jesus too. We learned to pray the Scriptures, we learned that God is faithful, and we learned that no other name but the name of Jesus is worthy of glory, power, and all praise.

The Saturday following Loretta's bone scan was uneventful. She only remembered that the next day was Danielle's nineteenth birthday and, once again, she would be celebrating away from us at college. We were grateful that her older brother would celebrate with her.

Loretta had complete assurance that the results from her latest scan would be good news. She was not preoccupied with it as she went about her daily life. At ten o'clock on Saturday night the phone rang and we were already in bed (very unusual for us) so I answered. Oncologist #2, the doubting doctor, was on the other end.

"Is Loretta there?" the doctor stammered. I handed the phone to my wife.

"Lady, you got your miracle! The hot spots are all gone! There are mere shadows where the cancer used to be. I hope you don't mind that I called you this late but you need to announce it to your church tomorrow morning."

He knew we had a praying church that believed in God and His miracles. We got down on our knees and thanked God for walking through the valley of the shadow of death with us. And then we called the children with the good news! Danielle said that when she got the news, she rushed up to the rooftop of her high-rise dormitory and sang, *How Great Thou Art* at the top of her lungs. Her roommate, Rachel, a faithful friend and prayer partner through the entire ordeal, sang along with her in joyous harmony.

When her brother Ben came over later to share the joy with her, they hugged and cried in front of her dorm and onlookers thought another Asbury College couple had just gotten engaged.

*"Praise the Lord, O my soul, and forget not all his benefits
— who forgives all your sins and heals all your diseases"*
(Psalm 103:2-4).

What a thrill for Loretta to share her testimony with the church body the following Sunday morning. She spoke briefly of our journey with cancer and how faithful God had been and then concluded with the news Oncologist #2 had given us the previous evening. When she said the words, "Lady, you got your miracle," most of the congregation stood up and raised their hands to God in praise. Some cried, others applauded and still others cheered. Our much-loved church family was not shocked, however, as this was the miracle they had been praying for. Their response was so beautiful to Loretta. Death had been all around us and the Lord had overridden it and proclaimed life. It was a glimpse of the raising of Lazarus in which, by His very presence, Jesus had proclaimed that where He is, death has no place.

"Bless the Lord, O my soul . . . who heals all my diseases"
(Psalm 103:1, 3, NKJV).

Loretta later testified, "The Word of God says that we are not to be anxious about the state of our bodies. We have trust in Him so we present our bodies a living sacrifice. The Word of God was the power that released the will of God in my life. I am the property of God and I am redeemed from the curse of cancer. His Word lives in me, even to the joints and marrow of my bones. I stand in full assurance that my healing has been secured through the blood of Christ. God's Word is a medicine to my bones!"

On Tuesday, October 3, Loretta kept her appointment with Oncologist #1. He walked into the examination room with his nurse, grinning from ear to ear. Looking at Loretta and me, he remarked, "Whatever you guys did, the National Cancer Research Foundation needs to be notified."

Loretta asked him, "Would you put in writing that this is a verifiable miracle?"

"Actually, I'll do you one better," he replied, lifting up the beautiful bone scan for us to look at. "I'm going to write an order for you to receive a copy of the before and after scans as well as a copy of the pathology report."

Looking at the scans, we could see that the Lord had taken away the hot spots. Once again we rejoiced in the Word of God that said, "I will not die but live, and will proclaim what the Lord has done" (Psalm 118:17).

For several weeks Loretta and I carried copies of those bone scans and shared them with everyone we met. Word spread, and to our surprise we received varied reactions within the Christian community, some of which were disconcerting. We were asked if a mistake might not have been made in the original diagnosis. Did the questioners believe that God could more easily forgive sins than heal the body?

Some seemed to be looking for a formula to follow so they could receive healing too. For instance, when they heard that Loretta and I had put Bible verses on the walls of our home, they tried that and other things we had shared in our testimony. Loretta was quick to point out that it was not what we did that healed her; it was faith in the character of God and His integrity to make good on His Word.

Because Danielle was a pre-med student at a Christian liberal arts college, she had asked her professors to pray for her mom. She took a copy of Loretta's bone scans to school with her and one of her professors put them on the overhead projector so the entire class could view the handiwork of God.

Some years later when I was preaching Fall Revival at Asbury College, Loretta had the opportunity to share her miracle with many of the staff who had prayed for her. She recalled a Valentine's Day prior to this and a rather curious gift I had given her. Danielle had gently informed me that another cookbook was not an appropriate gift, but she wasn't around to coach me on what was suitable. So I came home with a bundle of treasures: a beautiful, self-created card, thanking Loretta for being my only valentine for over twenty years; an "I Love You" coffee mug with a tiny white bear on it; a heart-shaped box of chocolates; and, most memorable, a plaque with her name on it with the words BATTLE MAIDEN inscribed under it.

To Loretta's knowledge she had never seen the meaning of her name on any plaque that Christian bookstores frequently sell. She responded to all the gifts with a gracious thank-you to me, but added that I could have left the name thing at the store. I quickly replied, "Hon, lighten up. It doesn't say battle-axe." I went on to tell her that someday she would be proud that her name meant something so militant.

Late one night the Lord made these words in Psalm 18:4-6 very real to Loretta:

> *"The cords of death entangled me; the torrents of destruction overwhelmed me. The cords of the grave coiled around me; the snares of death confronted me. In my distress I called to the Lord; I cried to my God for help. From his temple he heard my voice; my cry came before him, into his ears."*

The psalmist goes on to say in verses 16-19:

> *"He reached down from on high and took hold of me; he drew me out of deep waters. He rescued me from my powerful enemy . . . He brought me out into a spacious place; he rescued me because he delighted in me."*

Then comes the part that speaks of being militant, as recorded in verses 34-40:

> *"He trains my hands for battle; my arms can bend a bow of bronze. You give me your shield of victory, and your right hand sustains me; you stoop down to make me great. You broaden the path beneath me, so that my ankles do not turn. I pursued my enemies and overtook them; I did not turn back until they were destroyed. I crushed them so that they could not rise; they fell beneath my feet. You armed me with the strength of battle; you made my adversaries bow at my feet. You made my enemies turn their backs in flight, and I destroyed my foes."*

Lettie Cowman, one of the founders of One Mission Society, writes in her devotional, *Streams in the Desert*:

> *We are set to fight certain battles. We say we can never be victorious; that we can never conquer these enemies; but, as we enter the conflict, One comes and fights by our side, and through Him we are more than conquerors. If we had waited, trembling and fearing, for our Helper to come before we would join the battle, we should have waited in vain. . . . Press forward with bold confidence and take what is yours. "I have begun to give, begin to possess" (Deuteronomy 2:31).*

In the midst of our many blessings and also in the face of devastating news and challenges, God remained constant. And when we occasionally asked, "Why, God?" the words "battle maiden" and my gift to Loretta that Valentine's Day made sense.

Ben shares more reflections of our family and our journey through those days.

As I think about the home I grew up in, the word that most often comes to mind is "secure." During the early years, my parents did not make a lot of money but we never felt poor. We may not have had everything we wished for but we never wanted for anything.

During my teen years, when I came home after a tough day at school, I was aware of a great sense of peace filling our house. The world outside those walls didn't always make sense, but I was certain of my parents' love for me. I always knew that family was forever, and we had an unbreakable bond, regardless of what lay ahead.

This sense of security extended to what I had come to understand about God. I never doubted that my parents were faithful to God and to one another. Cognitively, I knew they were human and capable of error or sin, but it would not have crossed my mind to believe that either of them would deal with one another or anyone else in an ungodly way. To me, they were a perfect picture of what an idyllic Christian life and marriage should be.

Accompanying this image was a belief that God would always take care of those who lived faithfully. I had known Christians who had had tragedy befall them, but I somehow considered my parents to be exempt from such things. In my youthful mind, relationship with God had a mechanistic quality to it: God takes care of those who are faithful to Him. My parents were more committed to Christ than anyone I knew, so surely God would not allow us to face anything that we couldn't weather. We were secure in that house on Linden Street under God's protection.

As often happens when the assumptions of our youth collide with the realities of life, the time came when mine were shaken. I remember the day my parents walked up the stairs to my room on the third floor of our house to tell me about Mom's diagnosis. I especially remember Dad's eyes. I could tell he had been crying, and though it was not uncommon for me to see him with tears in his eyes after prayer, worship, or sometimes out of grief at a funeral, this was different. A sense of fear immediately gripped me because I could tell that he was trying very hard to be strong.

My dad had always had a bit of a John Wayne persona about him, seemingly an unassailable pillar of strength. But that day, the look on his face and the slight tremble in his voice revealed a hint of something different. I saw my dad shaken. I had never seen this before and at first it scared — and then angered — me. I was angry at cancer. I was angry at Satan. And then my anger turned toward God. Reflecting on it now, I understand where that anger came from: The security that I'd taken for granted my whole life up to that point was suddenly called into question.

I did my best to be strong and confident regarding Mom's healing, that day and in the days that followed. I recall thinking that this was one of those moments where I needed to grow up. My parents were facing a tough challenge, and at seventeen I was their oldest child. I didn't want them to have to worry about me and how I might be processing this assault on the security of our home.

I resolved to do my best not to cry in front of them. The problem was that a growing insecurity was starting to eat at me from the inside out. I was angry at God because, in my mind, He had not lived up to His side of the bargain. My security had been shaken, and when I was alone the fear was overwhelming. I'd weep for my mom, I'd weep for my dad, and while I believed that God was still with us (because my parents had not lost faith), I was unsure about what He wanted from us, from me in particular. Because God had allowed this to happen, my adolescent mind began to worry that if my mom wasn't rescued maybe it would be because I was the weak link in prayer. The fear was overpowering.

I don't remember exactly what was said that day. I remember my parents doing their best to reassure all of us that God was in control and that we would face this as a family. I recall my mom being remarkably serene. She seemed to me to be the strongest. I was particularly struck by her genuine concern primarily for us. Perhaps because I'm a male, my dad had always been the image of the primary protector, the invincible pillar we could stand behind and weather any storm, but that day, and in the days leading up to her surgery, I saw my mom in a new light. She had a strength that I'd never credited her for. She was always a woman of faith and had wonderful spirituality, but that day I saw a person of strength emerge, a warrior resolute and ready to go to battle on behalf of her family.

In the days ahead my dad leapt into action. There was much prayer at church for my mom. I remember Scripture verses on the subject of healing appearing all over the house. And I watched my parents draw closer together in the face of this oncoming storm. During our childhood my siblings and I often playfully ran down the steps only to find Mom and Dad kneeling in prayer together by the couch in the living room. We always retreated as quietly as possible because there was a sense of the holy in those moments. I seem to recall seeing them praying together more often than ever during this time. And that familiar image, along with their unfaltering faith, helped me begin to trust God again.

Ed and Loretta Williamson

CHAPTER 7

MORE REFLECTIONS

Facing cancer or any disease is a mountain to conquer. Faith is a relationship with Christ that grows into a trust that overcomes every situation and disease. Jesus is the light when we cannot see and by simply seeking the refuge offered by Him, we deposit a small amount of trust in Him who sees and knows everything. That trust grows and breaks up the mountain facing us. It shatters the darkness surrounding our mind and emotions so that we can walk with perfect peace. The cancer and pain are still present, but our faith is a trust-walk with God anchored in the faithfulness of His character.

Cancer does not determine our daily interchange with people and living life to the fullest. Once the smallest measure of trust is placed in Christ, we can say, "Lord, I do not understand Your ways, but You know the way for me."

Loretta and I did not have a significant amount of faith, but we knew what faith we had belonged in God's promises and His faithful character. The result was a path through the mountains we faced in our journey.

> *"I tell you the truth, if you have faith as small as a mustard seed, you can say to this mountain, 'Move from here to there,' and it will move. Nothing will be impossible for you"* (Matthew 17:20).

This verse about the mustard seed is very meaningful in understanding the power and process of faith. Jesus' disciples had failed in their attempts to drive out a demon that had cursed a young boy's life. The father had requested Jesus to have mercy on his son, explaining, "I brought him to your disciples and they could not heal him" (verse 16). Jesus' response was a stern rebuke for the disciples' lack of faith (verse 17) and then He rebuked the demon and healed the boy (verse 18). When the disciples went privately to Jesus and asked why they had failed (verse 19), Jesus responded with the lesson of the mustard seed.

This seed, generally considered the black mustard seed, was the smallest known at the time but it could grow up to nine feet into a large annual plant. It was not a garden plant but was found in outlying rural regions. The disciples were familiar with local vegetation and knew that the tiny seed would lodge itself inside the smallest of rock formations, grow into a tree, and break up the rocks in the process. Jesus was saying that the smallest amount of faith, just a tiny measure of it, could move mountains.

Loretta and I received a lot of advice and were given "methods" to use to receive our healing. We called them Christian "mantras" that seemed designed to convince, coerce, or manipulate God into healing her. These popular mantras are a shadow of the magical rites and formulas used in the Old Testament by the heathen to earn and/or demand the blessing of their pagan deities. The people of Israel were to reject these and worship the one true God who described Himself as holy and complete in Himself. It was to be a relationship with Yahweh designed for God to dwell in their midst without His holiness destroying them. The rituals and ceremonies of the Old Testament pointed to the Messiah, the Christ, who fulfilled all the promises for this personal relationship of the indwelling of the Holy Spirit in the heart of the believer.

Although well intended by sincere believers, the focus of these "methods" is wrong, because the teaching is in error. Faith is not a substance that can be collected and put into pill form, or into a syringe and injected into an individual. If that were the case, one could market a "faith pill" for those who feel they have weak faith that needs to be strengthened. Such thinking often is the result of ministries and/or healing crusades where individuals are the victims of emotional and manipulative methods. People are directed to follow certain steps to receive their healing, or told that they will experience healing along with some manifestation of the Holy Spirit (even sometimes sending them to the floor). The focus of our faith is never to be manifestations of the Spirit; rather, our focus should always be a single-minded, passionate love for Christ with the goal of having the mind of Christ and a heart that is cleansed of every rival to and hostility against God.

We came to the point of faith knowing that *to live is Christ, to die is gain.* This was the critical juncture in our journey toward healing. It was not an instantaneous experience or the result of an emotional service; rather, it was a process, the result of quiet time in personal communion with our Healer, Jesus Christ. The question of why some very spiritual people are healed and others die remains. In our ministry we have been with people who have come to this same juncture, questioning, "Lord, what is Your plan for me?"

In the hills of West Virginia lived a godly woman named Freda who contracted bone cancer. We anointed her with oil, read her scriptures relational to healing, and prayed with her regularly. At times she was in so much pain that we dared not touch her. Yet, in answer to prayer, the pain would subside for days at a time. We thought that surely one of these times the pain would subside permanently. One day as I visited her in the hospital and was about to pray for her, she interrupted me, "Don't pray for healing. The Lord showed me that He wants to take me home and I'm ready." She had reached the critical juncture, "Lord, what is Your plan for me?"

Another godly woman, Mrs. Teets, had a recurrence of cancer about the same time that Loretta experienced a healing. When offered a tape of Loretta's testimony, along with prayer, she sweetly replied that the Lord had already spoken to her heart. She knew her time on earth was complete, the Lord's purposes in her life had been fulfilled, and she was ready to go be with Him. Mrs. Teets was glorifying Christ and giving testimony to her personal relationship with Him.

Loretta and I were at the same juncture with many questions, even fears, regarding why godly people die and are not healed. But the only question we were earnestly seeking an answer to was, "Lord, what is Your plan for Loretta?" We became convinced through prayer and Bible reading that God's purposes for Loretta's life were not completed. Further, we were confident that her cancer was an assault against us and the ministry that God intended for us and our children. We did not arrive at this conclusion quickly as though hit by a bolt of lightning, but rather, it was a process that culminated in specific scriptures for both of us.

Once again Isaiah 41:12 became a bright light in the midst of the darkness and the battle we were fighting: *"Though you search for your enemies, you will not find them. Those who wage war against you will be as nothing at all."*

Those words became the Sword of the Spirit in our hands. Our enemy was cancer and God would make the power of the enemy as "nothing at all." There would come a day when they would "search for the enemy and not find him." From that point on I no longer petitioned the Lord to heal Loretta. I simply thanked Him and proclaimed these scriptures. At every meal these verses were quoted in a prayer of thanksgiving with a growing assurance based on the specific promise of God for our situation.

One of the "methods" proposed for us to use was to speak to the cancer and curse it. There was a spirit of infirmity that Jesus rebuked and the person was instantaneously healed. But most of the occurrences of healing in the New Testament were simple statements for healing. We placed our confidence in the only directive in Scripture for healing of the sick. It's recorded in James 5: the laying on of hands, anointing with oil, and the prayer of faith by the church elders.

We applied the scripture in James 4 where we are instructed to *submit yourselves to God, resist the devil and he will flee from you.* We prayed, we exalted Him in worship services, and submitted to the Word of God. At the same time, we dealt with organic evidence confirming that estrogen-fed cancer cells were in Loretta's body.

In our pastoral ministry, people experienced divine healing and heard testimonies of healing during worship services. It is in the context of the local church that God desires to manifest Himself. Praise and worship and Holy Communion should be a part of a local church's theology for the healing presence of Jesus. It was in worship and participation in the sacraments that Loretta and I received spiritual renewal and healing virtue for her body. There were times I observed her from the platform lifting her hands in worship to her Savior and Lord. I knew she was in pain in her shoulder and arm, but even though physical healing was not evident in her body, her spirit was renewed and her faith and trust in the Lord increased.

Convinced that Loretta's ministry was not complete and that her cancer was an attempt of the enemy to bring death to our ministry, we began to pray the scriptures. There were some scriptures that burned in my heart as a word from the Lord to us. Our prayers were based on the work of Jesus Christ and the fact that He is our Healer. We continued to pray Isaiah 41:12 over Loretta, specifically that every mutinous cancer cell in her body would come under the lordship of Jesus Christ and be rendered harmless to her in Jesus' name. There came a point that as we prayed this way, we would end with thanksgiving even though the doctors had not confirmed a healing.

I fought tremendous mental battles when I would envision Loretta in her casket, with our children and me being left alone. Was I lacking faith at that point? Was Loretta's healing in jeopardy because I was failing to meet the faith equation? No! I understood that it was a battle and, in my own frailty, I had to face these fears and have courage in the face of them. Just as God told Joshua three times to have courage in the face of entering the Promised Land and securing the promises, so I had to choose the promise over the anxiety and pictures of death. I could do this only because I knew where the source of her healing was anchored — not in me, but in Him.

The healing for Loretta was secured by the character and integrity of God and His Word. Since I understood that faith was not a substance that can evaporate in the heat of the spiritual battle, but a trust relationship with an unchanging God, I was not overcome with fear. The battles continued, but I didn't allow fear to find a permanent lodging in my heart. Whether healing occurred or not, God was in control and was leading us. That had become an unshakable reality in our hearts through Holy Scripture.

We saturated our minds with the Gospels, especially Mark's, and the accounts of healing and faith. My words became those of the father with the sick boy, "I believe. Help Thou my unbelief." It is never wrong to acknowledge the struggle, as it releases you from the false teaching of repeating the right formulas and mantras, while you are struggling with your belief and trust in God.

Hope in the Bible is not a mere possibility, but a reality. We speak of the "hope" of the resurrection of the body, not as a possibility, but rather a definite reality when Christ returns. Prayer and saturation in the Word of God allowed me to reaffirm what the Word said about Loretta's healing and our situation. This produced "hope." The battle in the mind subsided as the Scripture bolstered my faith and trust in my Savior as the Healer, regardless of the lab reports. The reality that the manifestation of her healing would occur was lodged in my heart. When I had battles, Loretta would be strong. When both of us were struggling, brothers and sisters in the church would encourage us with a scripture or a reassuring statement of faith.

When our church experienced a wounding of relationships, resulting in division that could have been the death of it — and

Loretta — we felt like King David when his son Absalom betrayed him. This was the worst of times for us. We were wounded and bleeding shepherds of an equally wounded and bleeding flock. We were facing a physical death sentence for Loretta, as well as a spiritual and emotional death sentence of the church we had birthed and nurtured for years. It was a time of hurt, anger, and confusion for all of us.

I had difficulty reconciling the rejection of the church and us by individuals in whom we had placed total trust. For the first time in thirty years of ministry, I had empathy for those pastors who leave the ministry feeling betrayed and wounded. Loretta and I had to work and pray that the hurt and anger would not take root in our hearts and result in resentment toward those whom we felt had wronged us. Above all, we had to extend forgiveness to every person and not allow a roadblock to be erected in the healing process for Loretta. Everything we had ever preached and taught had to be lived out in our lives.

It was Loretta who shared a Scripture truth from the life of Moses that gave us the patience and peace to endure. The Book of Numbers records that the leadership and integrity of Moses and his brother Aaron were challenged by Korah and his followers (16:3). The staff of Aaron was placed in the Ark of the Covenant, along with the staffs of other leadership, and in the morning only Aaron's staff had sprouted. Not only had it sprouted, but it had budded, blossomed and produced almonds (17:8). So God mightily reaffirmed the leadership and ministry of Moses and Aaron.

Loretta encouraged us by stating that there would be a "budding of Aaron's rod" in our ministry and that God would confirm His blessing. As we understood this principle of resting in the sovereignty and providence of God, we looked to Him to rectify all injustices, freeing us to forgive and refocus on our battle with cancer. Because stress is a natural accelerator of cancer (and many diseases), we wanted to keep Loretta's life as stress-free as possible. In the midst of what would be a deeply stressful time for any pastor, we experienced a sweet peace along with strong support from fellow believers.

The "budding of Aaron's rod" did occur. God positioned people to join our faculty, and school opened that fall only two weeks late. One of the most significant things Loretta and I did was assume the leadership of the youth group of three. Nathan has fond memories of the once bustling youth group meeting on Wednesday nights in the children's chapel. We met to pray that God would bring in new youth and we began to see answers to prayer. It was amazing! Every week new families came, families with teenagers who were teachable and hungry to learn about Jesus.

Nathan loved having Loretta and me lead the youth, and it is an honor to have your son think you're cool. Our house became the hangout and his friends knew that it was a safe place filled with genuine love and concern for them. Loretta had a beautiful gift for making others feel loved while at the same time challenging them. It was a special time because God was truly building the group; in fact, within just three months there were thirty young people meeting together.

We witnessed a return of strength to Loretta's body. The intense pain in her ribs subsided and I could hold her in my arms without hurting her. We believed the cancer was gone. It was time for the bone scans and we recalled the scripture from Isaiah 41:12 that we had made our own: *"Though they search for the enemy, they will not find him."* The medical report substantiated Loretta's healing from cancer. By Easter, the church attendance broke previous records, the children's ministry was growing, and within three years, we added a debt-free addition to the church.

The Word of God was our medicine for the physical and emotional healing . . . and continues to be (Proverbs 4:21-22).

In our Methodist tradition, every four years at the General Conference a General Superintendent is elected. In 1994 I was nominated for the position but I declined because I knew in my heart that I was not to leave Covenant at that time (and Nathan was still in high school). Loretta and I agreed that we needed to be open to God's will for our lives, so we allowed my nomination to stand for a vote at the 1998 General Conference. We had to put into practice what we had preached for so many years, even if it meant relocating.

In 1998, I was elected to the office of General Superintendent and this meant a move to Indianapolis, Indiana. Our walk with the Lord had always been to hold our lives with open hands, willing for God to add or remove positions of ministry.

Even though we knew we were moving in God's will and with His blessing, there were still some deep emotional tugs. I recall the day I had to knock on the front door of the church God had used me to plant because I no longer had a key. It was wrenching, yet in that moment it was deeply reaffirmed in my heart that Covenant was Christ's bride; it did not belong to Ed and Loretta Williamson. The ministry was never owned by us.

Pulling up roots in the mountains of West Virginia and moving to the flatland of Indianapolis caused us some sadness. But we also were energized and filled with great anticipation, righteous expectation, and a sense of deep peace. Peace always accompanies obedience to His leading.

CHAPTER 8

ANOTHER BEND
IN THE ROAD

My grandparents lived right off a narrow, twisting road bordered on each side with brush so thick and tall that in the summer visibility around the turns was almost completely obscured. To add to the danger, at points the road narrowed and when an oncoming car approached, one had to hug the ditch. My mother recalled that she would often blow the car horn when she approached some of the curves, fearful that she would meet another car — head-on.

In November 2001, six years after being declared totally clean of cancer, Loretta once again experienced symptoms. This reminded me of the road to my Grandpa Allen's house — not the end of the road, but just another bend in it. I knew, then, that we must continue to trust the Designer of the bends in life's road.

Pain returned at the incision site of Loretta's cancer, pain so intense that it kept her awake at night. One day, after a sleepless night, she experienced a "total emotional meltdown." She knew that God had healed her six years prior but this new pain stirred up doubts, and a heavy depression settled in on her.

"Why me? Why now?" Our first grandchild was due in a few weeks and our older son was scheduled to get married in three months. Such joyful events, yet so overshadowed by this latest crisis.

Other questions plagued her as well. Would this be the only grandchild she would live to see? Would she be bald for her son's wedding? She began to feel that perhaps this was a "sickness unto death" and that God's purposes for her life here were complete. She wondered if there were things she could have done differently — a sin or an unresolved problem. Or perhaps the stress of ministry caused the recurrence.

"Where is God right now? Why don't I have any faith today?" Question upon question found their way into her mind.

In the midst of our tears and discussions, God gave Loretta and me valuable insight. I was at a loss as to what to say or do to help her because, while I didn't express them aloud, I was grappling with the same questions as she. Yet, our faithful Father mercifully entered into our most excruciating moment to help us.

In my case, I was able to look at my wife and share encouraging words. "Loretta, nothing has changed from yesterday to today: God's grace is still over all. You certainly don't need to perform in order for God to deliver you from this new recurrence. And I just want to remind you that you don't have to be 'superwoman' every day."

Everything we receive from God, including healing, is undeserved and unmerited. I went on to encourage my wife by reminding her that God does not change and His character does not fluctuate, thus her healing is based on His grace and not her performance or faith formulas. We both realized that God wanted to deepen our relationship with Him. Loretta saturated her life with His Word and listened to worship music. A rest came into her heart and emotions when she contemplated the sovereignty of God. God had allowed this for His purposes and we were committed to living without worry about the days ahead of us.

During the month of December Loretta enjoyed days relatively free from pain, and she was able to go shopping with friends. One Sunday morning as she was worshiping at church, she was struck by the thought that God was with her before cancer struck. God was not taken by surprise by her circumstances. The truth of Isaiah 53:5 became real to her: *"He bore our infirmities and disease . . . and by His stripes we are healed."*

I busied myself by juicing about two pints of carrot juice a day for Loretta. I would pray over the juice, asking God to make its effects felt in her body and bring healing. We reaffirmed to each other that Jesus, and not cancer, was our focus. We resolved to use our mental faculties and energy to learn all we could about cancer, but our ultimate focus was to be upon Him.

The words from the ancient traditional Irish hymn *Be Thou My Vision* became our prayer.

> *Be Thou my vision, O Lord of my heart,*
> *Naught be all else to me, save that Thou art.*
> *Thou my best thought by day or by night,*
> *Waking or sleeping Thy presence my light.*

A pastor friend sent us a verse from a song by Karen Wheaton:

He'll do it again for you; He'll do it again.
Just take a look at where you are now and where you have
been.
Hasn't He always come through for you?
He's the same now as then.
You may not know how and you may not know when,
But, He'll do it again.

There were moments of great joy! Danielle's due date was drawing closer and Ben and Andrea's wedding date was moved up. Loretta felt that she had much to look forward to and she continually thanked God for His blessings on our family. Psalm 16 was a source of sweet comfort to her, especially verses 7 and 8:

"I will praise the Lord, who counsels me; even at night my
heart instructs me. . . . Because He is at my right hand, I
will not be shaken."

I was experiencing emotional turmoil and one evening I expressed to Loretta in a cracking voice, "I need you. You complete me. I don't want to continue in ministry without you." Loretta was quick to assure me that I would be able to carry on . . . without her. When she expressed this, I feared that she was going to remind me that God would give me a new wife after she was gone. I wanted no part of that. I wanted her to choose to live and I needed to hear in her voice a firm confidence that her ministry and life were not over.

As the time for some new pathology results drew closer, both Loretta and I found it difficult to focus on any one task for long. Loretta was questioning why a cancer that was medically verified to no longer exist could now resurface.

A few months before, she had experienced pain in her armpit so severe that she screamed aloud; in fact, these episodes often awakened her from a deep sleep. And then suddenly, the pain disappeared, and an indentation surfaced where the pain had been. Our doctor was as puzzled as we were and he promised to "keep an eye" on it.

Soon it was discovered that the cancer had eaten into the motor nerve and destroyed it, accounting for the cessation of pain. We had had no warning and we were plagued with questions: Should we have been more aggressive in getting a medical analysis earlier? Because we were so sure that it couldn't be cancer, could we have given the cancer time to invade the muscle tissue? And, most troublesome, did we fall into the "formula trap," depending on our learned pattern of dealing with cancer? After all, we reasoned, we had traveled all over the country testifying to Loretta's healing. Her response to all these new uncertainties was to get alone with God and hear from Him. She and I realized that we could not continue to live on past promises and "manna" given to us six years earlier. Our changeless God would meet our present need.

I began studying from the book of Joshua in preparation for team teaching with my son, Ben, who was now our pastor. I was especially encouraged by the words God spoke to Joshua, "Be strong and courageous." Courage in the face of circumstances over which one has no control is so important. The Promised Land was already Joshua's to possess and he and the people must have the courage to face down the obstacles in their path. I saw that it was the same for salvation and physical healing. Grace has provided for them and faith must be exercised to possess them. We began to seek God for fresh promises from His Word.

We recognized that one struggles to balance the role of medicine and the role of faith for physical healing. We certainly didn't want our ministry to end with the epithet: Trusted Only in Physicians. My prayer was, "Lord, I am determined, with the enabling power of the Holy Spirit, to have the courage and strength to allow Your Word to establish my faith, as opposed to being swayed by medical diagnoses. At the same time, we need Your wisdom and guidance in using medical science to extend Loretta's life and bring healing by Your hand."

I still felt intense pain at the possibility of Loretta not being by my side in ministry. I was convinced that her death would be a victory for the enemy by shortening her ministry before God was finished with it. I wanted it to be God's call for Loretta to "come home," and not cancer that would finalize her days on earth.

Loretta, too, was firm in her belief that cancer would not determine her years, God would. She had always loved the story she had heard about Bill Bright, the founder of Campus Crusade for Christ. When he accepted Christ into his life, he took a blank piece of paper and signed his name at the bottom. And then he raised it up to the Lord and said, "Jesus, I want You to fill in the details." That was Loretta's desire, too. She never wanted to be wealthy or famous, she just wanted to be a servant of the Lord for as long as He allowed her to be.

Loretta was convinced that God heals today and she also acknowledged that He doesn't work the same in each case. She was a great admirer of Pastor Rick Warren and identified with his wife, Kay, who also had battled breast cancer. When Warren's book *The Purpose Driven Life* became a runaway best-seller, he said, "I didn't know what to do with all that money, so I sought the Lord and He spoke to me from His Word. First, I asked my church not to pay me any more salary and then I returned the entire salary I had received in the previous twenty-four years." The lesson he was conveying was that you must surrender the good things in life as well as the bad.

An excerpt from *The Purpose Driven Life* was especially meaningful to Loretta.

> *One day my heart is going to stop and that will be the end of my body, but not the end of me. When your life is fully surrendered to God He determines when your heart will stop, not cancer, not your heart, not anything else. The reason the Christian has trials is because God is more interested in your character than He is in your comfort. He's more interested in making your life holy rather than happy. You can focus on God's purpose for your life or you can focus on your problems. If you focus on your problems you're going to be centered on "my problem, my issues, my pain." If you focus on others and God's Word, it's the easiest way to get well.*

Loretta was able to say, "All I know is that God owns my life. He bought it with the price of the cross. He paid the penalty for my sin and my indifference all those years I rejected Him. Oh, maybe not outright, but I rejected Him by giving Him only one day a week. I gave Him Sunday mornings when He wanted all of me all the time. We will have a zillion years in eternity to spend with Him. We're here for only one speck of time and we embrace it like it is forever. It's not! Our choice is to follow Christ and spend eternity with Him or reject Christ and spend eternity without Him. The secret to endurance is to remember that your pain is temporary, and your reward eternal."

During her last five years, when the physicians told her that all they could use going forward were experimental drugs, Loretta lovingly thanked them, but replied, "I am more concerned about my quality of life than I am about the quantity. I am leaving that in God's hands."

Although in pain and experiencing various infirmities, Loretta gathered the ladies in the community to our home for a book club. She chose a Christian biography and used it as a format to share her faith and discuss how to live a complete life. Danielle and I chuckled as we observed her using the "generic" book club to try to be incognito while sharing the gospel. All the ladies in the neighborhood already knew her faith and loved her.

In the last three years of her life Loretta had to limit her travels, but she discipled her nieces in Massachusetts and West Virginia and other young women to whom she and I had ministered at Covenant. They would email questions to her and she would respond; actually, it became a fruitful ministry. Loretta set up appropriate books for them to read jointly and then had them report on a chapter every week. And when nieces and nephews visited for a week, Loretta used a part of each day to take them through Pastor Jim Cymbala's video series on prayer. The family observed her body weakening, but her passion for people to know Christ and become mature disciples never diminished.

CHAPTER 9

OUR LAST CHRISTMAS

Loretta and I always believed that the Lord would show us when she was nearing the end of her journey on this earth. During the 2012 Advent Season, we both became aware that this most likely was our last Christmas together. We didn't tell our children that we sensed Loretta's death was near and so no effort was made on their part to be with us for a "last Christmas." Loretta and I celebrated it, as well as each other, alone.

Once we determined that this was our final Christmas together, we doubled down on our studies about heaven. We read and reread the book of Revelation between Christmas and the end of May.

Loretta enjoyed reading books about heaven written by Randy Alcorn, and together we discussed his book about a new heaven and a new earth merging as one. C.S. Lewis' writings were also favorites, especially *The Chronicles of Narnia*. Lewis' view of heaven was that the new heaven and the new earth were on a grander scale, beyond our natural comprehension, resembling the landscape and skyline of the present earth.

Christianity is the only religion in the world where God comes to us offering a relationship with Himself. All other religions are efforts to work out a path to God for His acceptance, striving to earn merits and rewards. In Christianity God came to us in Jesus the Christ, dying on the cross for our sins and transforming us for a relationship with Him. In Christianity God is our friend, our heavenly Father, but in other religions their god is far off, unreachable, demanding. So it is not surprising that at the end of time, God creates a new heaven that comes to transform what we know now into a new earth.

Orthodox Christianity holds the Bible's interpretation of a literal heaven. Every person is a living soul with the possibility of having a living relationship with the Creator. After death, life is not a vacuum or some kind of nirvana in a meaningless existence. Rather, it is wonderful beyond what we can grasp, a beautiful new earth in a perfect relationship with our Creator. When Jesus said in John 14:3, "I go and prepare a place for you," He was talking about a literal place.

The Apostle Paul said, "To be absent from the body (our earthly physical body upon death) is to be present with the Lord" (2 Corinthians 5:8). Loretta and I discussed what this fulfilled relationship with the Lord would be like, since she would be free of sin and a cancerous body. We found comfort knowing she would no longer be in pain and would have reached "the prize" of eternal life with God (see Philippians 1:21-23).

Gospel songs such as *When We all Get to Heaven* convey the thought that upon death, we are going somewhere from here. As just stated, for the Christian, dying means that we "will be with the Lord." This is what we need to call the "intermediate heaven," to use the phrase of Alcorn and some of the church fathers. It is not a place for a second chance for entrance into heaven; rather, it is for those who have received the forgiveness of their sins by trust in Christ on this present earth, but await the final consummation of all things and the resurrection of the dead in Christ. When the dead in Christ are raised, those who have been promoted to the intermediate heaven will receive a new resurrected body likened to the body of the risen Lord Jesus.

The main point in understanding the Scripture about heaven is grasping the fact that we do not "go up there" into the heaven but "heaven comes down to earth," forming a new heaven and new earth as one reality (see Revelation 21:1-3). Peter says this earth as we know it will be destroyed and "burn with fervent heat" (2 Peter 3:7-10). What we now know and experience will be destroyed at the coming of the Lord Jesus Christ (1 Thessalonians 4:13-17). The final outcome will be a new heaven and a new earth where we will work and dwell together.

In the gospels we see that following the resurrection, the disciples recognized Jesus Christ when He appeared without time boundaries and the limitation of space. Christ would appear in the room and converse with the disciples, or appear on Galilee's seashore preparing a meal for those in the fishing boat. Likewise, we will know one another in heaven and visit with family and friends. In this intermediate heaven we can assume from Scripture that the saints are aware of the events on earth. Hebrews calls this the "cloud of witnesses" overlooking the evolving history of humankind and God's unfolding purposes.

Have you been in a hospital and suddenly heard a lullaby being played over the speaker system? That is the signal that a new baby has just been born there. The Bible says that the angels rejoice whenever a person receives Christ as his or her personal Savior, experiencing the forgiveness of sins. There is an awareness of what is happening on earth by those in the intermediate heaven.

Loretta and I realized that she would be aware of what was happening in my life, and in the lives of our children and grandchildren. As I reflect on this time, I believe this understanding about heaven was such a definite reality to both of us that Loretta was enabled to make more rational suggestions and observations.

She began the New Year on a roll — a woman with a mission. She was determined to find a good mate for me and she made a list of beautiful Christian women who she thought would be suitable. At one point I had to insist that she stop this, although, true to her character, she persisted — and occasionally word of her "schemes" leaked out to me.

I had upgraded Loretta's original engagement diamond the Christmas before and, as frugal as she was, she prized it. She had a private conversation with Danielle, making her promise to tell me that I was to sell the diamond ring and use the money for a ring for my new bride when that day came. When I found out about this, I rejected the idea outright. Danielle, as our only daughter, would get her mother's ring! If and when God sent the right woman along for me, I would take care of a ring for her.

Loretta and I were upfront with each other about our emotions, and discussed the transition both of us would face. She often prayed aloud for the future Mrs. Williamson because she held to a firm conviction that God had prepared a mate who would come alongside me in my ministry.

Several years earlier we had created a "bucket list." A cruise from Rome to Amsterdam had been given to us so that was easily checked off. However, as inviting as traveling and seeing new sights was, we realized that more urgent matters needed to be added to the list. Loretta knew and loved many individuals who didn't know Christ. Some were relatives who were deeply religious but lacked a personal relationship with Jesus. We created a list that followed our pattern of many years of praying for individuals and nations on specific days of the week.

During the winter and spring months, we experienced a gradual letting go of each other — alternating between love and clinging to one another. At a Saturday evening church service during Holy Week, while singing resurrection hymns Loretta was forced to hold on to me for support. With tears streaming down my face, I watched my beloved wife stand with her free arm raised, singing, "He arose, He arose, Jesus Christ arose." I pictured her standing before her risen Lord, cancer free and pure from all sin. As total peace filled my heart, I said to God, "She was always Yours first, and now I release her back to You."

This was a memorable experience for me, and only in Loretta's final weeks of life did I mention it to her. Yet, I found it very difficult to release her physically from my life. I would profoundly miss her touch and our sharing of life together. God's grace enabled me to open my heart to Him in worship and receive strength for the days ahead.

Loretta's bone pain began to gradually increase and medication adjustments were necessary to make her comfortable. Our denomination, of which I am still General Superintendent, held its annual conference in April with pastors and laypeople gathering in Lake Junaluska, North Carolina. Loretta attended with me, experiencing only one bad day. I had to caution well-meaning friends to refrain from hugging her, as her bones were brittle and painful. Loretta loved hearing God's Word, especially the Old Testament, and worshiping along with the pastors at the sessions. She and I both knew that this would be her last Journey Conference, as they were called.

The drive back to our home in Indianapolis was a seven-hour trip. On the way, Loretta spent an hour on the phone sharing Christ with a young man who had been a kindergarten student of hers years earlier. She never missed an opportunity to share Christ's love, even in her weakened state of health.

We now had several grandchildren and they were waiting for us when we returned home. Loretta played some games with them but the exertion took its toll on her body. The next day, a Saturday, she was in such horrible pain that she needed stronger medication. That very day Danielle was receiving her master's degree from Indiana Wesleyan University but Loretta was too weak to attend the ceremonies so I stayed with her and we watched a live streaming of the event.

By Monday, Loretta's pain had increased, and although I didn't want to leave her alone, I had to make a quick trip to my office to retrieve some items. While I was out, Loretta reached me by phone. Rushing home, I found her collapsed on the bathroom floor, and lying down beside her, I told her that we were no longer able to manage her pain — it was time to call hospice. She agreed, and even though we both knew that this day was inevitable, it seemed to arrive so suddenly.

A hospice nurse came that very afternoon and she brought wonderful ministry into our lives. She was knowledgeable and kind and at one time when Loretta resisted taking "too much" of the strong painkillers for fear of becoming addicted, the nurse just smiled and gently reminded her, "No, that won't happen." She further explained to Loretta that without them, her quality of life would be substantially diminished.

The hospice professionals projected that Loretta probably had two months of life left. Because some cancer deaths are such protracted ordeals, Loretta and I had prayed that she would be spared that. Within two weeks, with Loretta's decline apparent, the hospice nurse changed her projection. (Loretta went home to be with the Lord five weeks from the time hospice came into our home to minister to us.)

During those final weeks, our family realized that we were losing the Loretta we knew and loved. She enjoyed sitting on the deck in the sunlight while her grandchildren played and talked to her. Danielle and even the grandchildren, who lived nearby, ministered wonderfully to Loretta and me during this period.

For most cancer patients, increasing pain is accompanied by a high level of anxiety; consequently, Loretta's anti-anxiety drugs were administered right along with her pain medications. It should be understood that this apprehension has nothing to do with one's relationship with God. One specific focal point of Loretta's anxiety centered around her portable oxygen; if it wasn't right beside her, she would panic.

Loretta revived her bucket list of people she wanted to share Christ with — she called it "playing her cancer card." She busied herself calling her nieces and nephews and, after assuring them of her love for them, she gave them an affirming message of God's love and faithfulness, explaining that He had a marvelous plan for their lives.

She wanted to share with one particular nephew, but by this time she had declined to the point that she was having trouble keeping her thoughts together well enough for articulate expression. The children and I were afraid that it was too late for her to have a meaningful conversation but our son put the call through anyway. To everyone's amazement, Loretta lucidly shared the love of God and her testimony with this special nephew. That was the last time she was able to converse so fluently — and it was also the last check on her bucket list.

Leah, one of our daughters-in-law, has a calling to children's ministry. One afternoon she sat down with Loretta and peppered her with questions about ministry to children and rearing children in general. Loretta had such a wealth of information and wisdom, and people were amazed at how beautifully she was able to share with Leah. Only one week later she was not able to communicate so cogently.

I asked our children to relay some of their recollections of those last days of Loretta's life. Nathan, our younger son, and now a pastor, had this to say:

> *Dad, I remember lots of things, but what stands out is the last deep conversation I had with her before everything started to go downhill fast. I asked Mom how you guys met and the circumstances of her being kicked out of the house by her parents after she chose to follow Jesus. She told me lots of things I had never heard before. Then she told me that she was proud of me and of what God was doing and was going to do through me. She prayed for me, and I for*

her, and then we held hands and laughed and cried in her bed.

Another memory is of singing praise songs with her. At one point she stopped me and said, "You won't believe me, but all the words you're singing I am seeing on the ceiling of my bedroom in beautiful colors going up to the sky." I remember how her fear would leave her when we talked about heaven, Jesus, or eternity. Her eyes would light up and peace would wash over her.

Every time I came back to visit her that last month of her life, I would walk into her room and she would say, "Praise the Lord!" I especially remember the last time I visited with her, which was a Sunday, and, although she couldn't talk, she did respond when I told her of God's work in church that day.

I had attended the Journey Conference in April along with you and Mom. We were between sessions and I went for a walk, as my heart was hurting with the burdens of ministry. I ended up in your room. Mom was so tired she could hardly get out of bed. I shared my heart with her and she affirmed me and cried with me. I told her how much I needed her and that I didn't want her to ever leave. She reassured me again by telling me about her weaknesses and her constant need to depend on Jesus. She encouraged me by telling me that Jesus saw and knew my heart — and that was what should give me worth and value. I really miss those talks.

I received a sweet assurance from the Lord after Mom passed. He reminded me of the passage of Scripture where Jesus told His disciples that it was better that He go so that the Comforter would come. That passage took on new meaning for me once Mom was gone. What was better than having Jesus in person minister to me? Now, without my mother as my "go-to" support, I was forced to depend on the Holy Spirit, to trust Jesus for myself, with the power of the Holy Spirit. I more fully understand how Mom could be who she was. It wasn't that she was superhuman; it was that she was a mere human who had learned that real strength lies in surrender to and reliance on Jesus. That was the gift her passing gave to me. No longer does my wisdom and strength come from Loretta first, then the Lord. It was better for me that she left so that the Comforter could come and be my rock.

To make Loretta more comfortable I had to secure a hospital bed. Thinking it would take at least a day to process the order and that Loretta and I could share our bed one more night, I placed the order. To my surprise (and dismay), the bed arrived within two hours. For the remaining weeks of Loretta's life I slept on the couch right beside her bed so I could administer her medications during the night.

One night prior to moving into the hospital bed, Loretta had asked me if I had seen "that man" outside our bedroom window. I replied that I hadn't, but asked her if the man's presence instilled peace or fear in her. She replied that he brought her peace. Later, when she was situated in her hospital bed, she observed this same man and had the same peaceful response to him.

On the evening before Loretta passed from this life, she said to me, "The man is here in the room."

I asked her what he was doing, and she replied, "He is slowly walking back and forth."

"Loretta, I think he has come for you and heaven is near."

I was reminded that the Bible speaks of angels, ministering spirits assigned to each of us. In her last hours on earth, with Christian music playing, it was as if her steady gaze penetrated the ceiling into eternity. In this atmosphere of peace, my Loretta entered into Paradise on June 2, 2013.

Loretta was insistent that her body be dedicated for research and the remains cremated. Her thought was that God had done miraculous things in her physical body and there might be something in her cellular structure that would move science toward a cure of cancer.

We had already determined not to have the memorial celebration service in Indiana, but at home in West Virginia at Covenant. Our son Nathan was now the pastor and he had upgraded the media technology in the church so we could show the service online. A few years earlier, Loretta had spoken at the *Race for the Cure* weekend at our church in Greenwood, Indiana. She always "knocked it out of the park," although she was never convinced of that fact. I had arranged for her presentation to be recorded and we used portions of that DVD at the memorial service. In that way, Loretta actually preached her own memorial service.

The family gathered the night before the service to listen to the clips that Nathan had chosen to use. When we heard her voice and saw her on the monitors, our emotions overwhelmed us. Likewise, the next day those attending the memorial were not prepared to hear Loretta speaking to them and they had similar emotional responses. We all loved her and missed her. The service was powerful as Loretta shared personally about our journey with cancer; our sons Ben and Nathan and her sister Denise also shared their testimonies.

An unexpected development was that the family could not experience full closure because we did not receive her earthly remains for a year. When we finally had the graveside ceremony, it was brief but it had its impact. All the grandchildren were there and I knelt and spoke to them about the powerful work of grace in their "Mémère" and affirmed their memories of her. I was able to point to their great-grandfather's grave and share how the gospel transferred down through generations, impacting them with the spiritual heritage that was theirs to possess.

One very meaningful song from the memorial was *In Christ Alone*.

In Christ alone my hope is found
He is my light, my strength, my song;
This Cornerstone, this solid ground
Firm through the fiercest drought and storm.
What heights of love, what depths of peace
When fears are stilled, when strivings cease!
My Comforter, my All in All
Here in the love of Christ I stand.

In Christ alone, who took on flesh
Fullness of God in helpless babe.
This gift of love and righteousness
Scorned by the ones He came to save:

Till on that cross as Jesus died,
The wrath of God was satisfied.
For every sin on Him was laid;
Here in the death of Christ I live!

No guilt in life, no fear in death,
This is the power of Christ in me;
From life's first cry to final breath,
Jesus commands my destiny.
No power of hell, no scheme of man
Can ever pluck me from His hand,
Till He returns or calls me home,
Here in the power of Christ I'll stand.

By Keith Getty and Stuart Townend

I am frequently asked, "When did you lose your wife?" I gently and humbly respond that I didn't lose her; I know where she lives. I am mindful that Christianity is the only religion whose Founder left an empty tomb. Jesus rose from the dead after having died on the cross for all sins and those who accept that will spend eternity with their Lord once this journey ends.

Looking back on Loretta's more than twenty-year struggle with cancer, our shared testimony was, "We never would have volunteered for this battle with cancer, but we would not trade it for another journey in light of what God worked in and through our lives for His glory."

I can now confidently proclaim, "Cancer was never victorious, although it ravaged Loretta's body. Grace was always greater for every footstep of our journey together." I am equally confident that whatever path God leads me down, the challenges are not hindrances but platforms from which to testify to God's love, grace, and truth in power. We lived with cancer every day, but we did not allow cancer to govern our daily lives.

CHAPTER 10

THE BATTLE IS THE LORD'S

God does heal the physical bodies of people today just as He healed the sick throughout biblical history. The healing ministry of the New Testament is centered in the local church, with elders of the church anointing with oil and praying the prayer of faith (James 5:13-18).

The first healing is the experience of conversion and the spiritual new birth of the person. This includes the acknowledgement of being a sinner and asking God's provision for the forgiveness of sins, made possible by the blood of Christ on the cross. Eternal life, salvation, is the gift of God that replaces any religious performance that earns this salvation.

"I am a sinner, forgive me of my sins, change my heart to be like Christ's," is the prayer for healing. This begins the faith/trust relationship with God. As we see in Genesis 12, Abraham was a "friend of God." God in Christ is your greatest friend, but greater still is your heavenly Father. Even if your earthly father was cruel, your heavenly Father is good and extends to you a relationship you can trust and be secure in. I encourage you to place your trust in Christ, be baptized, and begin the journey to the life you were born to live.

In 1 Samuel 13, King Saul is a picture of a man of partial obedience, impatient and willful, and this led to the breakdown of a genuine personal relationship with God. When David and Saul each were caught in sin, the difference between the two men was the depth of their relationship with Yahweh. Saul made excuses (verses 11-12) and David repented (Psalm 51). In verse 12, Saul says, *"I have not sought the Lord's favor,"* even though he had seven days to wait for Samuel. This is important to remember when praying for healing.

Saul's faith never became personal; he never sought God on his own. He believed only when the battle was led by Samuel or David, which was demonstrated in the story of Goliath: *"Go, and the Lord be with you"* (1 Samuel 17:37). David conquered Goliath because of his relationship with God; Saul failed because his relationship with God was fractured.

David burned with passion when he saw the army of God in fear.

> *"Who is this uncircumcised Philistine that he should defy the armies of the living God?"* (1 Samuel 17:26).

King Saul tried to put David in his armor but when David strapped it on and tried walking around in it, he said, *"I cannot go in these …because I am not used to them"* (verse 39). This is an important principle: God and man fight battles differently. God owns the battle, God chooses the weapons, and God fights the battle for us. Because of his personal relationship with God, David could respond to the negative predictions of doom and death with resolve:

"The Lord who delivered me from the paw of the lion and the paw of the bear will deliver me from the hand of this Philistine" (verse 37).

So what did God choose? He chose smooth rocks from the creek bed, a slingshot, and a shepherd boy's trained arm to kill the giant.

What will God use to slay your giant? Only in the interpersonal relationship of quiet moments will you determine whether it is an instantaneous or gradual healing using anointing oil and prayer, or a result of medical procedures. Don't become impatient and get ahead of God; He runs the battle and is never taken by surprise.

How is it when it is just you and God? Loretta had a lot of human support, but it was in the inner citadel of her mind and heart that faith and trust grew. She learned that there is no other name, no other tower to run into than the presence (face) of God.

How is it for you when the prophet doesn't show up, as in Saul's case, and there seems to be no good news? Will you wallow in pity and fear or, like Hezekiah, will you roll over in bed and seek God about your illness (see Isaiah 38)? It is much easier to seek God's hand of power than it is to seek His face for relationship.

Let's look at the story of King Asa's lack of faith in his later years and how he trusted only in the doctors. In the early years of his forty-one-year reign as king of Judah, he was a righteous king who relied on the Lord for his success. He is described as doing *"what was good and right in the eyes of the Lord his God"* (2 Chronicles 14:2).

But later in life, Asa was afflicted with a serious disease in his feet and he did not turn to the Lord.

"Though his disease was severe, even in his illness he did not seek help from the Lord, but only from the physicians" (2 Chronicles 16:12).

Somewhere along the line Asa became self-sufficient and proud, and neglected his relationship with God. He did not seek Him even when he was desperately ill.

"For the eyes of the Lord range throughout the earth to strengthen those whose hearts are fully committed to Him" (16:9).

If you are committed to seeking God with all of your heart and are teachable like King David, then you are God's candidate. He is seeking you out right now in your sickness and He needs to give you His strength.

The Apostle Paul promises us the ministry of the Holy Spirit *"who dwells in us to quicken our physical bodies"* (Romans 8:11). Paul reminds us that the same power that raised Jesus bodily from the dead lives in us to bring physical strength to our bodies. This passage of Scripture was quoted daily at our mealtimes for Loretta's physical body. Good nutrition, lots of carrot juice, prayer, and the promises of God resulted in physical strength returning to her body.

Guidance and healing are based on the promises of God found in the Bible. These promises reflect God's integrity and character. We must accept, believe, and trust that what He says in the Word, He will do. The person seeking healing and comfort must start with the Bible and the promises of God. Faith and trust are allowed to grow through times of quality prayer, participating in the sacrament of the Lord's Supper, communing with the Lord, and saturating the mind with Scripture. Ask the Holy Spirit to empower you to rely upon God's Word for your faith; ask Him to keep you from becoming distracted by circumstances, pain, or medical diagnoses.

Find rest for your soul in the sovereign will of God and ask Him specifically if His plans and purposes for your life have been fulfilled. Ask the Holy Spirit to enlighten your mind with specific passages of Scripture that apply immediately to your circumstances and ignite fresh faith and trust within your heart.

If you and your family know your journey is truly ending, make it the most blessed transition into heaven as possible with your family. As a married couple, one of you will have his or her earthly journey end first, reaching the goal of being with Christ. In the midst of pain medications and medical care, love each other and witness to those in your circle of influence. I opened the memorial celebration for Loretta with these words: "Cancer is dead in Loretta's body, but Loretta is not dead."

Declare the works of God in your life and to those around you as a witness to your faith.

The battle is the Lord's! There is **no other name.**

Ed and Loretta Williamson

EPILOGUE

As you have read, Loretta prayed that God would send me a wife after she went on to heaven, and it is my joy to share with you that her prayers have been answered. At the urging of my niece Julie, I made contact with a lovely, highly accomplished, godly woman named Gilda. Her husband James went to be with the Lord over 13 years ago and he had asked the Lord to send her a new partner.

Gilda and I found that we are very similar and compatible, and after several months we pursued a relationship. My three children and her two children were involved with us from the first contact, praying for us and encouraging us. They lovingly traveled the emotional and yet positive journey to our decision to marry. We sealed our commitment to one another in a private wedding ceremony in June 2015, two years after Loretta died. As Gilda and I now serve God together, we have been surrounded by the loving support of friends and family.

Benjamin, our firstborn, was born in Beverly, Massachusetts, north of Boston, just as I entered Gordon-Conwell Theological Seminary. Ben graduated from Asbury College, now Asbury University, with a degree in secondary education and a Bible major. Following his graduation from Wesley Seminary with a Master of Divinity, he served in the Evangelical Methodist denomination as a pastor and church planter. Today he serves as Associate Professor of Bible and Church History at Circleville Christian University and is earning his PhD from Dayton University School of Theology.

Danielle pursued a degree in biology secondary education with a minor in chemistry. She was awarded the Biology Student of the Year award and graduated summa cum laude from Asbury College. She became a teacher like her mother and has taught in public and Christian schools. She also completed her master's degree in curriculum and instruction through Indiana Weslyan University. During Loretta's medical struggles, Danielle read the lab reports and explained them to us while she was still in school. She and her family later lived near us in Indianapolis and she was one of the greatest supports of her mother during the last five years of her life.

In the early morning hours a little over three years after Loretta's death, Danielle was reading the final draft of this book. She came across her mom's application of Isaiah 54:13 and 14 *(All your sons will be taught by the Lord, and great will be your children's peace. In righteousness you will be established: tyranny will be far from you;*

you will have nothing to fear. Terror will be far removed; it will not come near you), and she felt as if Loretta were in the room sharing it with her. In Danielle's own words:

> *I had been concerned about my own children, about how they were assimilating their faith through their loss, and about what "teaching" they might be receiving when they were not with me. I felt the Lord's presence in a strong way and these verses directly addressed my fears on many levels.*
>
> *I felt as though I had shared my heart with my mom, and she had a verse to share with me that directly reached the heart of the issue. Because that is what she had done on so many different occasions throughout my life. Leave it to her to not let something small like death keep her from ministering to me.*

Nathan graduated from Asbury College in Media Communication with a triple emphasis in production, multimedia, and performance. He attended two Olympics and could have had a career in media because of his strong gifts in that area. However, he had the anointing of God on his life, and the call to full-time ministry could not be denied. Nathan graduated with a Master of Divinity from Wesley Seminary and today he is pastor of Covenant Evangelical Methodist Church in Morgantown, West Virginia, the church Loretta and I started.

Ed and Loretta on their wedding day, May 8, 1971, in Brooklyn, New York.

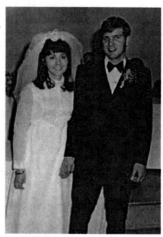

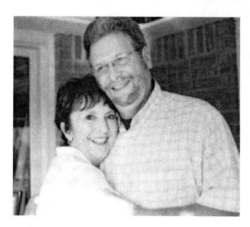

At home in Indianapolis, Ed and Loretta were partners in love and in ministry (2002).

Ed and Loretta vacationing in New Hampshire, enjoying the Atlantic Ocean (2009).

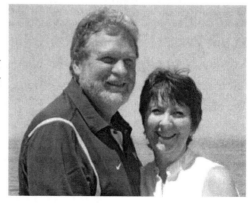

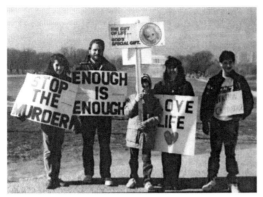

*The Williamson family,
March for Life,
Washington, DC (1989)*

*First business card
of CURE Corps.*

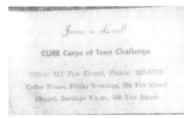

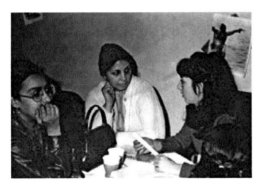

*Loretta ministering to
young women on Fox Street
through CURE Corps, the
ministry outreach started by
David Wilkerson where she
and Ed met.*

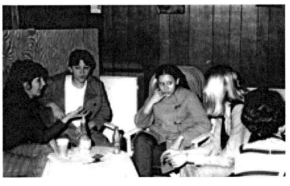

Ed and Loretta Williamson

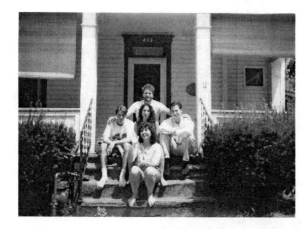

*The Williamsons
at home in
Morgantown, WV
(1990).*

*Ed and Loretta with
their children, Ben,
Danielle and Nathan
(Christmas 2011).*

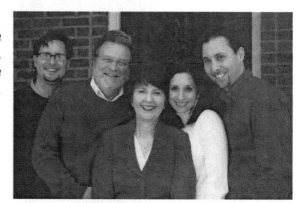

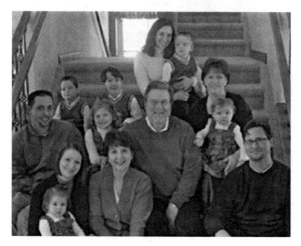

*Ed and Loretta with
their children and
grandchildren
(Christmas 2011).*

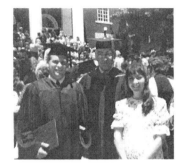

Dr. Lowell Roberts, with Ed and Loretta at Ed's graduation from Asbury College, 1974. Loretta was pregnant with our firstborn, Benjamin.

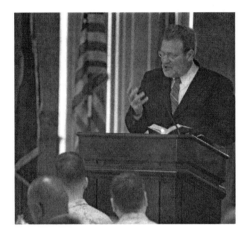

Dr. Ed Williamson at the National Day of Prayer, Camp Lejeune Marine Base, Jacksonville, NC (2008).

Danielle's graduation from Indiana Wesleyan University, just one month before Loretta's promotion to heaven (2013).

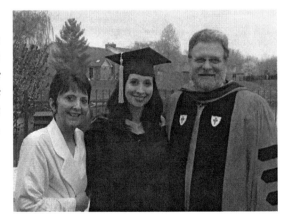

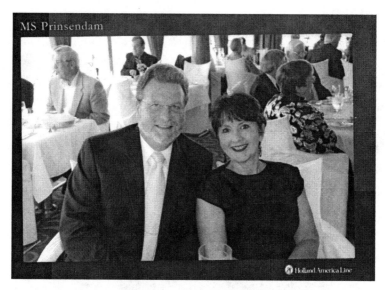

Our dream cruise from Rome to Amsterdam (2010).

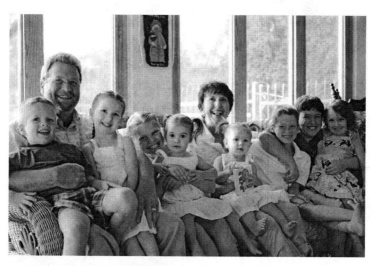

Loretta was always thrilled to be with our grandchildren.
L-R: Joseph, Emma, Kaylee, Ava, Hannah, Elijah, David, and
Rebecca. (Photo by Laura Yurs, 2012)

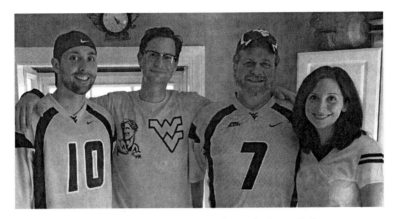

Nathan, Ben and Danielle with their dad
on a WVU game day (2014).

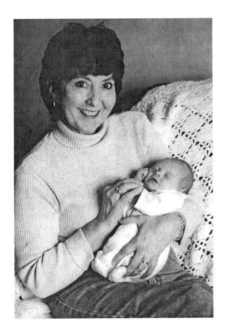

A blessing she was unsure she would ever see.
Loretta holding her first grandchild,
Kaylee, in 2002.

ABOUT THE AUTHORS

A native of Parkersburg, West Virginia, Dr. Ed Williamson knew he was called to ministry when he was only a teenager. He followed that vision to Teen Challenge, a ministry to drug addicts in New York City, where he met Loretta. She became his wife and loving partner in ministry for forty-two years.

An accomplished teacher, Loretta earned a BS in Elementary Education with an emphasis in Special Education from Fitchburg State Univery (Massachusetts) and an MA in Early Education from West Virginia University.

Ed earned his BA from Asbury University, his MRE from Gordon-Conwell Theological Seminary, MDiv from Asbury Theological Seminary, and his DMin from Boston University School of Theology.

Together Ed and Loretta planted Covenant Evangelical Methodist Church in Morgantown, WV, serving there for fourteen years. As forerunners of expanding daycare facilities into early childhood education schools, they also founded Covenant Christian School. Beginning as a preschool, under the leadership of Loretta CCS became a thriving, fully functioning K-8 Christian school which continues to influence generations for Christ.

Ed now lives in Indianapolis, IN, along with his wife Gilda, and continues to serve as International General Superintendent of the Evangelical Methodist Church denomination.

To order additional copies of this book:

Website: http://noothername2013.com

Facebook: No Other Name 2013

Evangelical Methodist Church International Headquarters: (317) 780-8017

For more information, write to us at noothername2013@gmail.com

Contributions from the sale of this book will be made to the Loretta Williamson Endowment for student scholarships at Covenant Christian School.

CPSIA information can be obtained
at www.ICGtesting.com
Printed in the USA
FFOW04n2057120817
38790FF